Celiac Disease Cookbook for Kids

Safe and Nutritious Gluten-free Recipes for Kids
(With Colorful Pictures)

Dr. Kaswui Dawui

All rights reserved.

Reserved rights. Without the publisher's prior written consent, no part of this publication may be copied, distributed, or transmitted in any way, including by photocopying, recording, or other electronic or mechanical methods, with the exception of brief quotations used in critical reviews and other non-commercial uses allowed by copyright law. Write to the publisher if you want to request permission.
copyright © Kaswui Dawui

TABLE OF CONTENTS

INTRODUCTION
What is Celiac Disease?
Why Do Children with Celiac Disease Need a Special Cookbook?
How to Prepare and Eat Gluten-Free

CHAPTER 2: BREAKFAST RECIPES
Gluten-Free Oatmeal with Fresh Fruit and Honey
Gluten-Free Pancakes with Blueberries and Maple Syrup
Gluten-Free Waffles with Bananas and Whipped Cream
Gluten-Free Crepes with Strawberries and Nutella
Gluten-Free French Toast with Cinnamon and Powdered Sugar
Gluten-Free Bagels with Cream Cheese and Smoked Salmon
Gluten-Free Breakfast Muffins with Apples and Cinnamon
Gluten-Free Yogurt Parfait with Granola and Berries
Gluten-Free Breakfast Smoothie with Bananas, Peanut Butter, and Almond Milk
Gluten-Free Quinoa Porridge with Sliced Almonds and Honey
Egg, bacon, and cheese breakfast pizza made without gluten
Gluten-Free Frittata with Spinach and Feta Cheese
Gluten-Free Breakfast Quesadilla with Scrambled Eggs and Cheese

Gluten-Free Breakfast Sandwich with Ham, Egg, and Cheese on a Gluten-Free English Muffin
Gluten-Free Breakfast Bowl with Brown Rice, Scrambled Eggs, and Veggies
CHAPTER 3:RECIPES FOR LUNCH
Turkey and Cheese Roll-ups
Grilled Chicken Skewers
Zucchini Noodles with Marinara Sauce
Gluten-free Chicken Nuggets
Lettuce wraps with turkey
Quinoa Salad
Grilled Cheese Sandwich on Gluten-Free Bread
Tuna Salad
Gluten-Free Pizza
Roasted Vegetable Salad
Gluten-Free Mac and Cheese
Turkey and Avocado Wrap
Grilled Salmon Skewers
Vegetable Stir-Fry
CHAPTER 4:RECIPE FOR DINNER
Baked Chicken Tenders with Sweet Potato Fries
Gluten-free Pizza with a Cauliflower Crust and Toppings of Choice
Grilled Salmon with Quinoa and Roasted Vegetables
Tacos made with Corn Tortillas, Ground Beef, and Avocado
Turkey and Mashed Sweet Potatoes

Baked Ziti made with gluten-free pasta and ground beef or turkey
Stuffed Bell Peppers with Ground Chicken and Quinoa
Grilled Chicken Skewers with Vegetables and Rice
Beef Stir-Fry with Broccoli and Gluten-Free Tamari Sauce
Chicken Parmesan made with Gluten-Free Bread Crumbs
Cauliflower Fried Rice with Shrimp or Chicken
Slow Cooker Chicken and Vegetable Soup with Gluten-Free Noodles
Baked Salmon Cakes with Roasted Sweet Potato Wedges
Sloppy Joes made with Gluten-Free Buns and Ground Turkey or Beef
Vegetable and Quinoa Stuffed Portobello Mushrooms

CHAPTER 5:RECIPES FOR A SNACK AND SIDE DISH
Baked Sweet Potato Fries
Roasted Chickpeas
Cucumber and Tomato Salad
Guacamole
Caprese Skewers
Hummus and Veggies
Popcorn with Nutritional Yeast
Baked Buffalo Cauliflower Bites
Deviled Eggs
Spinach and Artichoke Dip
Sweet and Spicy Mixed Nuts

Pita Chips and Tzatziki
Bruschetta
Baked Zucchini Fries
Stuffed Mushrooms
CHAPTER 6:DESSERT RECIPES
Classic Chocolate Chip Cookies
Fudgy Brownies
Vanilla Bean Cupcakes with Buttercream Frosting
Lemon Bars
Cinnamon Rolls with Cream Cheese Frosting
Strawberry Shortcake
Blueberry Crisp
Chocolate Mousse
Apple Pie with Crumb Topping
Peach Cobbler
Carrot Cake with Cream Cheese Frosting
Raspberry Cheesecake Bars
Chocolate Lava Cake
Banana Bread with Walnuts
Tiramisu
CONCLUSION

INTRODUCTION

When Emily was diagnosed with Celiac disease, it felt like the whole world was turned upside down. The little girl who once loved nothing more than devouring slices of pizza and biting into freshly baked bread suddenly found herself unable to eat anything containing gluten. Her body had become her enemy, attacking itself every time she consumed even the slightest trace of the protein.

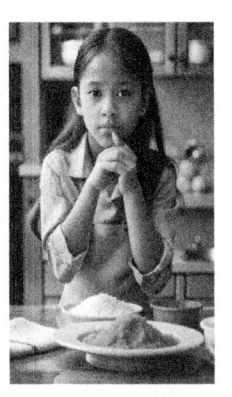

At first, Emily struggled to come to terms with her diagnosis. She felt angry and resentful, unable to understand why this happened. But her parents were determined to help her. They sought out the best dietitians, read every book they could find on Celiac disease, and spent countless hours experimenting in the kitchen, searching for gluten-free recipes that their daughter would love.

It was a long and challenging journey, filled with tears and frustration. Emily missed her old life, the carefree days when she could eat whatever she wanted without a second thought. But slowly, as she adapted to her new way of life, something incredible began to happen. Her body started to heal.

It wasn't an overnight process. There were setbacks and challenges along the way. But Emily's parents never gave up, and neither did she. She learned to love the new foods that were now a part of her life, discovering the joy of eating quinoa, buckwheat, and millet. She found ways to socialize with her friends without feeling left out, bringing her gluten-free snacks to parties and picnics.

As time went on, Emily's health continued to improve. Her stomach aches disappeared, and she had more energy than ever before. And one day, as she sat down to a delicious gluten-free meal with her family, she realized that she had been given a precious gift. She had learned to take care of her body, to nourish it with the foods that it needed, and in doing so, she had found a new way of living that was truly mind-blowing.

CHAPTER 1

Here you will find a cookbook for children with celiac disease. With Celiac disease, which alters how the body responds to gluten, this cookbook is intended to support children. Several common foods, such as wheat, barley, and rye, contain the protein known as gluten. When a person with Celiac disease consumes gluten, their immune system reacts by harming the lining of their small intestine, which can result in a variety of symptoms and long-term health issues.

Knowing how difficult it may be to locate items that are safe to eat if you or a member of your family has Celiac disease. The ability to prepare gluten-free meals at home is crucial because a lot of processed goods and restaurant cuisine contain gluten. The goal of this cookbook is to assist families with Celiac illness in overcoming the difficulties associated with following a gluten-free diet while still allowing for the enjoyment of scrumptious and nourishing meals and snacks.

You can find a range of dishes in this cookbook that is designed especially for children with Celiac disease. These recipes are created to be simple to prepare and delicious to consume. They include gluten-free items that are safe for persons with Celiac disease to eat. You will have many options for each meal because we have included recipes for breakfast, lunch, supper, snacks, and desserts.

Before we dive into the recipes, we'll provide some background on what Celiac disease is and why it's important to follow a gluten-free diet if you have this condition. We'll also offer tips for cooking and eating gluten-free, including how to read food labels, how to make substitutions in recipes, and how to avoid cross-contamination in the kitchen.

Living with Celiac disease can be challenging, but with the right tools and resources, it's possible to lead a healthy and happy life. We hope this cookbook will be a valuable resource for you and your family as you navigate the world of gluten-free cooking and eating.

What is Celiac Disease?

When gluten is consumed, the body's immune system develops celiac disease, causing the small intestine to be mistakenly attacked by the body. As a thickening or binder, processed foods frequently contain gluten, a protein that is present in wheat, barley, and rye. Gluten causes an immunological reaction in people with Celiac disease that destroys the lining of the small intestine, which can result in a variety of symptoms and long-term health issues.

Damage to the small intestine may result in nutritional malabsorption, which may result in several symptoms, such as fatigue, bloating, abdominal pain, diarrhea, and weight loss. The development and growth of children with Celiac disease can be delayed. As the small intestine continues to deteriorate, there is a chance that other health issues, like osteoporosis, anemia, infertility, and some forms of cancer, will also become more likely to manifest.

It runs in families since celiac disease is a genetic illness. The prevalence of celiac disease is thought to be one in 100 persons worldwide, however, many cases go unrecognized. A stringent gluten-free diet, which entails shunning any foods containing gluten, is the only cure for celiac disease. As many typical foods, such as bread, spaghetti, cereal, and baked goods include gluten, doing this can be difficult. But those with Celiac disease can still lead active, meaningful lives if they receive the correct information and support.

Why Do Children with Celiac Disease Need a Special Cookbook?

To control their illness, kids with Celiac disease must first adhere to a rigorous gluten-free diet. This entails abstaining from all gluten-containing meals, which can be difficult for kids who are accustomed to eating things like bread, pizza, and pasta. Finding kid-friendly gluten-free foods can be challenging for parents, particularly when dining out or attending social gatherings. By offering recipes that are both safe and delectable, a dedicated cookbook for children with Celiac disease helps ease the transition to a gluten-free diet.

The nutritional requirements of kids with Celiac disease are very special. Gluten can cause small intestine damage, which can impair the body's ability to absorb vital vitamins and minerals. Making ensuring that children are getting enough of these nutrients through their diet is crucial because this can affect their growth and development. Recipes that are not only gluten-free but also nutrient-rich for children with Celiac disease can be found in a specific cookbook created for this population of youngsters.

In addition, many children with Celiac disease often have other dietary allergies or sensitivities. For instance, some kids may have allergies to dairy, soy, or eggs, which can make it even harder to locate wholesome food. A specialized cookbook for children with Celiac disease can include recipes that take into consideration these other dietary limitations, giving families a larger range of options.

The value of a gluten-free diet can also be conveyed to youngsters and their families through the use of a special cookbook designed for children with celiac disease. It can offer guidance on how to understand food labels, prevent cross-contamination in the kitchen, and prepare safe and delectable gluten-free meals and snacks. Families can feel more confident managing their child's Celiac illness and enhancing their general health and well-being by arming them with this knowledge.

How to Prepare and Eat Gluten-Free

1. Know what foods contain gluten and which ones are safe to eat before you start to properly prepare and consume gluten-free food. It's crucial to carefully read labels and search for gluten-free certifications when shopping because wheat, barley, rye, and some oats all contain gluten. It's also crucial to educate yourself about cross-contamination and how to prevent it in your kitchen.

2. Think ahead: When consuming no gluten, meal preparation is crucial. To make sure you have all the items you need, plan your meals in advance and develop a grocery list. When you're hungry

and rushed for time, this can help you resist the urge to eat foods that contain gluten.

3. Use gluten-free alternatives: A variety of gluten-free alternatives are offered, including gluten-free bread, pasta, and flour. Find what works best for you by experimenting with various brands and types. The flavor and texture of some gluten-free products may differ from those of their gluten-containing equivalents, so be ready to modify your cooking and baking appropriately.

4. Concentrate on entire foods: One of the greatest methods to make sure you're getting all the nutrients you need when following a gluten-free diet is to concentrate on whole, unprocessed foods. Fruits, vegetables, lean proteins, nuts, and seeds are all included in this. These foods are naturally gluten-free and rich in fiber, vitamins, and minerals.

5. Be inventive: Although preparing and consuming food free of gluten can be difficult, it can also present a chance for culinary innovation. Explore new culinary creations and play around with flavor profiles and ingredients. The fact that

gluten-free meals can be tasty and filling may surprise you.

6. Avoid cross-contamination: Cross-contamination can occur when gluten-containing foods come into contact with gluten-free foods. This can happen in your kitchen, at restaurants, or even at the grocery store. To avoid cross-contamination, use separate cutting boards, utensils, and cookware for gluten-free foods. Additionally, be cautious when eating out and always communicate your dietary needs to the server or chef.

7. Be patient: Following a gluten-free diet can be a big adjustment, and it can take time to get used to. Be patient with yourself and don't be too hard on yourself if you make mistakes or slip up. With time and practice, cooking and eating gluten-free will become second nature.

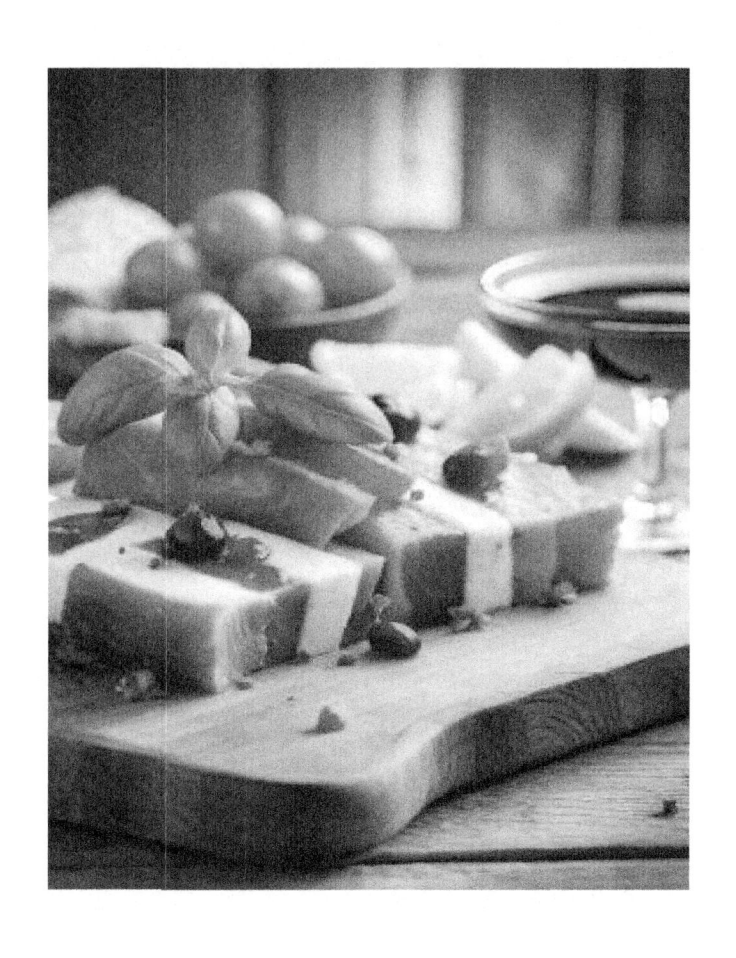

CHAPTER 2

BREAKFAST RECIPES

Breakfast is frequently seen as the most significant meal of the day, and children with Celiac disease must begin the day with a healthy, gluten-free meal. Here are some recipes for kid-friendly gluten-free breakfast foods:

Gluten-Free Oatmeal with Fresh Fruit and Honey

Ingredients:

- 1 cup gluten-free rolled oats
- 2 cups water
- 1/4 teaspoon salt
- Fresh fruit (such as sliced bananas, strawberries, blueberries, or raspberries)
- Honey or maple syrup, to taste

Instructions:

1. Bring the water and salt to a boil in a small saucepan.

2. Turn the heat down to medium-low after adding the gluten-free rolled oats.
3. When the oats are soft and the mixture has thickened, simmer the oatmeal for 10 to 12 minutes while stirring occasionally.

4. Oatmeal should be taken from the heat and allowed to cool somewhat.

5. Add fresh fruit to the dishes after spooning the oatmeal into them.

6. Honey or maple syrup can be drizzled over the fruit and cereal.

7. Enjoy your wonderful gluten-free oats with fresh fruit and honey when served hot!

Gluten-Free Pancakes with Blueberries and Maple Syrup

Ingredients:

- 1 cup gluten-free all-purpose flour

- 2 tablespoons granulated sugar

- 1 teaspoon baking powder
- 1/2 teaspoon baking soda
- 1/4 teaspoon salt
- 1 cup buttermilk
- 1 large egg
- 2 tablespoons melted butter or oil
- 1/2 cup fresh blueberries
- Maple syrup, for serving

Instructions:

1. The gluten-free all-purpose flour, granulated sugar, baking powder, baking soda, and salt should all be thoroughly blended in a medium basin.

2. The melted butter or oil, buttermilk, and eggs should all be thoroughly mixed in a separate basin.

3. When the batter is smooth, add the wet ingredients and whisk them together.

4. Then, include the fresh blueberries.

5. Over medium heat, preheat a nonstick skillet or griddle.

6. Pour 1/4 cup of batter into the skillet for each pancake and cook for 2 to 3 minutes, or until bubbles appear on the surface.

7. It takes around 1-2 minutes to cook the pancake from the other side until it is golden brown.

8. Do the same thing with the remaining batter.

9. Enjoy your delectable gluten-free pancakes with blueberries by serving them hot with maple syrup.

Gluten-Free Waffles with Bananas and Whipped Cream

Ingredients:

- 2 cups gluten-free all-purpose flour
- 2 tablespoons granulated sugar
- 2 teaspoons baking powder
- 1/2 teaspoon baking soda

- 1/4 teaspoon salt
- 1 1/2 cups milk
- 2 large eggs
- 1/4 cup melted butter or oil
- 1 ripe banana, sliced
- Whipped cream, for serving

Instructions:

1. All-purpose gluten-free flour, sugar, baking soda, baking powder, and salt should be thoroughly blended in a medium basin.

2. The milk, eggs, and melted butter or oil should all be thoroughly mixed in a separate basin.

3. Mix the batter until it is smooth after adding the wet components to the dry ones.

4. Spray nonstick cooking spray into a waffle machine and preheat.

5. Pour enough batter to completely cover the waffle maker's surface, then cook the waffles as directed by the manufacturer.

6. Continue by using the remaining batter.

7. Warm waffles should be served with whipped cream and sliced bananas.

Gluten-Free Crepes with Strawberries and Nutella

Ingredients:

- 1 cup gluten-free all-purpose flour
- 2 tablespoons granulated sugar
- 1/4 teaspoon salt
- 1 1/4 cups milk
- 2 large eggs
- 2 tablespoons melted butter or oil
- Strawberries, sliced
- Nutella, for serving

Instructions:

1. The granulated sugar, salt, and gluten-free all-purpose flour should all be thoroughly blended in a medium bowl.

2. Whisk the milk, eggs, and melted butter or oil together thoroughly in a another basin.

3. When the batter is smooth, add the wet ingredients and whisk them together.

4. Spray non-stick cooking spray into a non-stick skillet and heat over medium-low.

5. Pour enough batter to completely cover the skillet's surface, then swirl the pan to spread the batter out into a thin layer.

6. For about 1-2 minutes, or until the edges begin to brown, cook the crepe.

7. For an additional 1-2 minutes, flip the crepe over and cook the other side.

8. Do the same thing with the remaining batter.

9. With cut strawberries, serve the crepes hot.

Gluten-Free French Toast with Cinnamon and Powdered Sugar

Ingredients:

- 6 slices gluten-free bread
- 2 large eggs

- 1/2 cup milk

- 1/2 teaspoon ground cinnamon

- 1/2 teaspoon vanilla extract

- 2 tablespoons butter or oil

- Powdered sugar, for serving

Instructions:

1. Eggs, milk, cinnamon powder, and vanilla extract should all be thoroughly blended in a shallow basin.

2. Make sure to uniformly coat both sides of each piece of gluten-free bread before dipping it into the egg mixture.

3. In a nonstick skillet over medium heat, melt the butter or oil.

4. Cook the coated bread slices in the skillet for two to three minutes per side, or until golden brown on both sides.

5. Repeat with the remaining slices of bread.

6. Add powdered sugar to the French toast before serving it hot.

Gluten-Free Bagels with Cream Cheese and Smoked Salmon

Ingredients:

- 4 gluten-free bagels
- 4 ounces cream cheese, softened
- 4 ounces smoked salmon
- 1/4 cup red onion, sliced
- 1/4 cup capers
- Fresh dill, chopped

Instructions:

1. Set the oven's temperature to 375°F (190°C).
2. The gluten-free bagels are cut in half, then put on a baking sheet.
3. The bagels should bake for 5-7 minutes, or until only barely browned, in the preheated oven.
4. Spread a liberal amount of softened cream cheese on each half of the bagel.

5. Add some smoked salmon slices to the top of each half of the bagel.

6. Slices of red onion, capers, and finely chopped fresh dill should be added to each bagel half.

7. While they are still warm, serve the gluten-free bagels with cream cheese and smoked salmon.

Gluten-Free Breakfast Muffins with Apples and Cinnamon

Ingredients:

- 2 cups gluten-free all-purpose flour
- 2 teaspoons baking powder
- 1/2 teaspoon baking soda
- 1/2 teaspoon salt
- 1 teaspoon ground cinnamon
- 1/2 cup unsalted butter, softened
- 1/2 cup granulated sugar

- 2 large eggs

- 1 cup unsweetened applesauce

- 1 teaspoon vanilla extract

Instructions:

1. Achieve a 375°F (190°C) oven temperature.

2. Put paper liners in a muffin tray.

3. Mix the baking powder, baking soda, salt, and ground cinnamon in a medium bowl with the gluten-free flour.

4. The softened butter and granulated sugar should be combined in another big bowl and beaten until frothy.

5. Add the eggs one at a time by beating.

6. Stir in the vanilla essence and applesauce until well mixed.

7. Add the dry ingredients a little at a time while mixing the wet components until just mixed.

8. In the prepared muffin cups, distribute the batter evenly.

9. In the preheated oven, bake the muffins for 20 to 25 minutes, or until a toothpick inserted in the center comes out clean.

10. After the muffins have cooled in the pan for a few minutes, then transfer them to a wire rack to cool completely.

Gluten-Free Yogurt Parfait with Granola and Berries

Ingredients:

- 2 cups gluten-free granola
- 2 cups vanilla Greek yogurt
- 2 cups mixed berries (such as strawberries, blueberries, and raspberries)

Instructions:

1. Layer the vanilla Greek yogurt, mixed berries, and gluten-free granola in a little bowl or container.

2. Up till the top of the bowl or jar, repeat the layering process.

3. Immediately serve the yogurt parfait without gluten, or chill until ready to serve.

Gluten-Free Breakfast Smoothie with Bananas, Peanut Butter, and Almond Milk

Ingredients:

- 2 ripe bananas
- 2 tablespoons gluten-free peanut butter
- 1 cup unsweetened almond milk
- 1/2 teaspoon ground cinnamon
- 1/2 teaspoon vanilla extract
- 1 cup ice cubes

Instructions:

1. The ripe bananas, gluten-free peanut butter, unsweetened almond milk, ground cinnamon, and vanilla extract should all be combined in a blender.

2. The mixture should be smooth.

3. Blend in the ice cubes after you've added them.

4. The gluten-free morning smoothie should be poured into a glass and served right away.

Gluten-Free Quinoa Porridge with Sliced Almonds and Honey

Ingredients:

- 1 cup quinoa
- 2 cups water
- 1/2 teaspoon ground cinnamon
- 1/4 teaspoon ground nutmeg
- 1/4 teaspoon salt
- 1/2 cup unsweetened almond milk
- 1/4 cup sliced almonds
- 2 tablespoons honey

Instructions:

1. Quinoa should be well rinsed with cold water that is running.

2. Quinoa, water, cinnamon, nutmeg, and salt should all be combined in a medium saucepan.

3. Over medium-high heat, bring the combination to a boil.
4. When the quinoa is soft and the liquid has been absorbed, reduce the heat to low and simmer the mixture, covered, for 15 to 20 minutes.

5. Add the almond milk without sugar, honey, and almond slices.

6. Serve the gluten-free quinoa porridge right away after dividing it evenly among the bowls.

Egg, bacon, and cheese breakfast pizza made without gluten

Ingredients:

- 1 gluten-free crust for pizza
- 50 ml of tomato sauce
- Shredded mozzarella cheese in a cup

- 4-slices of cooked and crumbled gluten-free bacon

- Four big eggs

- To taste, add salt and pepper.

- fresh parsley, chopped, as a garnish

Instructions:

1. Set the oven's temperature to 425°F (220°C).

2. Pizza crust devoid of gluten should be put on a baking sheet covered with parchment paper.

3. With a 1-inch border around the edges, cover the pizza crust with the tomato sauce.

4. Over the tomato sauce, strew mozzarella cheese crumbles.

5. Add the cooked and crumbled gluten-free bacon on the pizza.

6. Spread the eggs out evenly over the pizza after carefully cracking each one.

7. Add salt and pepper to taste to the eggs.

8. The gluten-free breakfast pizza should be baked in the preheated oven for 10 to 15 minutes, or

until the cheese is melted and bubbling and the eggs are cooked to your preference.

9. If preferred, top the pizza with freshly cut parsley before serving.

Gluten-Free Frittata with Spinach and Feta Cheese

Ingredients:

- 6 large eggs
- 1/4 cup unsweetened almond milk
- 1/4 teaspoon salt
- 1/4 teaspoon black pepper
- 1 tablespoon olive oil
- 2 cups baby spinach leaves
- 1/2 cup crumbled feta cheese

Instructions:

1. Heat the broiler.

2. Eggs, unsweetened almond milk, salt, and black pepper should all be combined in a medium bowl.

3. In a sizable oven-safe skillet, warm the olive oil over medium heat.

4. Baby spinach leaves should be added and cooked for 2 to 3 minutes, until wilted.

5. The spinach leaves in the skillet will be covered with the egg mixture.

6. Over the top of the egg mixture, evenly distribute the feta cheese crumbles.

7. On the burner, cook the frittata for 5 to 6 minutes, or until the bottom is lightly browned and the sides are firm.

8. Place the skillet under the preheated broiler for two to three minutes, or until the top is gently browned and the eggs are completely set.

9. Remove the skillet from the broiler and let the frittata cool for a few minutes before slicing and serving.

Gluten-Free Breakfast Quesadilla with Scrambled Eggs and Cheese

Ingredients:

- 2 gluten-free tortillas
- 4 large eggs, scrambled
- 1/2 cup shredded cheddar cheese
- Salt and pepper, to taste
- 1 tablespoon olive oil
- Salsa and sour cream, for serving (optional)

Instructions:

1. Large skillet heated to medium heat.
2. Olive oil is added, then the skillet is thoroughly coated by swirling it around.
3. The skillet should include one gluten-free tortilla.
4. Scrambled eggs and cheddar cheese are sprinkled on top of the tortilla.
5. Add salt and pepper, as desired, to the eggs and cheese.

6. The other gluten-free tortilla should be positioned on top of the eggs and cheese.

7. Cook the quesadilla for 2 to 3 minutes on each side, until the cheese is melted and the tortillas are crisp and gently browned.

8. With salsa and sour cream, if preferred, serve the gluten-free breakfast quesadilla in wedges.

Gluten-Free Breakfast Sandwich with Ham, Egg, and Cheese on a Gluten-Free English Muffin

Ingredients:

- 2 gluten-free English muffins, split and toasted
- 4 thin slices of gluten-free ham
- 4 large eggs, scrambled
- 4 slices cheddar cheese
- Salt and pepper, to taste

Instructions:

1. Heat the broiler.

2. On a baking sheet covered with parchment paper, spread out the toasted gluten-free English muffin halves.

3. Slices of gluten-free ham should be placed on top of each muffin half.

4. Scrambled eggs should be placed on top of the ham.

5. Add salt and pepper to taste while seasoning the eggs.

6. On top of the scrambled eggs, place a slice of cheddar cheese.

7. The gluten-free breakfast sandwiches should be placed under the preheated broiler for two to three minutes, or until the cheese is melted and bubbling.

8. Serve the gluten-free breakfast sandwiches right away.

Gluten-Free Breakfast Bowl with Brown Rice, Scrambled Eggs, and Veggies

Ingredients:

- 1 cup cooked brown rice

- 4 large eggs, scrambled
- 1 tablespoon olive oil
- 1/2 cup diced bell peppers
- 1/2 cup diced onions
- 1/2 cup sliced mushrooms
- Salt and pepper, to taste

Instructions:

1. Heat the broiler.
2. The toasted gluten-free English muffin halves should be distributed across a parchment-lined baking sheet.
3. Topping each muffin half with a slice of gluten-free ham is recommended.
4. On top of the ham, you should put scrambled eggs.
5. As you season the eggs, add salt and pepper as desired.
6. Add a slice of cheddar cheese to the scrambled eggs.

7. It is recommended to broil the gluten-free breakfast sandwiches for two to three minutes, or until the cheese is melted and bubbling.

8. Sandwiches made without gluten should be served right away.

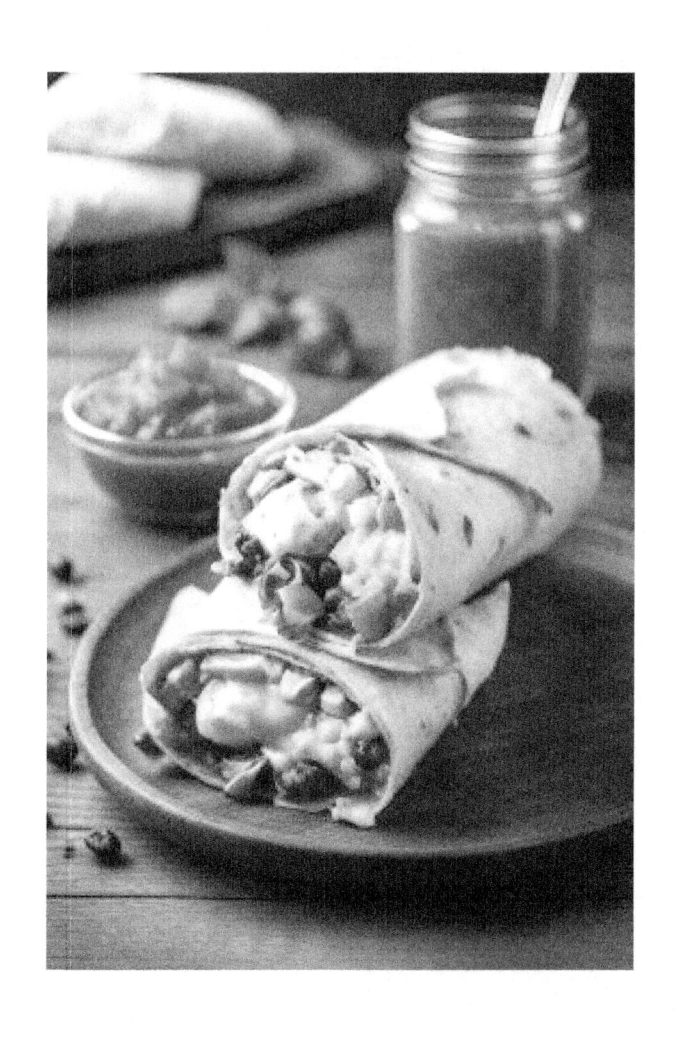

CHAPTER 3

LUNCH RECIPES

Finding gluten-free options for lunch might be difficult, but kids with Celiac disease can enjoy a variety of delectable and filling gluten-free meals with a little imagination. These recipes for lunch are suggested:

Turkey and Cheese Roll-ups

Ingredients:

- Sliced turkey breast
- Sliced cheese (choose a gluten-free variety)
- Toothpicks

Instructions:

1. On a cutting board, arrange a flat slice of turkey breast.
2. On top of the turkey, place a slice of cheese.

3. Cheese and turkey are firmly rolled.

4. Put a toothpick in to hold.

5. Continue until you have as many roll-ups as you like.

6. Serve plain or with the gluten-free dipping sauce of your child's choice.

Grilled Chicken Skewers

Ingredients:

- 1 pound chicken breast, cut into strips
- 1/4 cup gluten-free soy sauce
- 1/4 cup honey
- 1 tablespoon sesame oil
- 1 tablespoon minced garlic
- 1 tablespoon grated ginger
- Skewers

Instructions:

1. The honey, sesame oil, minced garlic, and grated ginger should all be combined in a bowl with the gluten-free soy sauce.

2. As soon as the chicken strips are added, toss them in the marinade to coat.

3. At least 30 minutes or up to 2 hours should pass before covering and chilling food.

4. The heat should be set to medium-high on the grill or grill pan.

5. Stick the skewers with the marinated chicken strips.

6. For the chicken skewers to be fully cooked, grill them for 5-7 minutes on each side.

7. Serve hot as an accompaniment to a salad or vegetable, or as a side dish with your child's preferred gluten-free dipping sauce.

Zucchini Noodles with Marinara Sauce
Ingredients:

- 3-4 medium zucchinis
- 2 tablespoons olive oil
- 1 small onion, chopped
- 2 cloves garlic, minced
- 1 can (14 oz) gluten-free diced tomatoes
- 1 teaspoon dried basil
- Salt and pepper, to taste

Instructions:

1. Use a spiralizer to create noodles out of the zucchini.

2. Melt the olive oil in a large skillet over medium heat.

3. To the skillet, add the chopped onion and the minced garlic, and cook for about 5 minutes, or until the onion is tender.

4. Stir together the salt, pepper, dry basil, diced tomatoes, and add to the skillet.

5. Turn the heat down to low and simmer the sauce for 10 to 15 minutes.

6. Cook the zucchini noodles for 1 to 2 minutes, or until soft, in a separate pot of boiling water while the sauce is simmering.

7. Drain the noodles, then combine with the marinara.

8. Enjoy a hot serving!

Gluten-free Chicken Nuggets:

Ingredients:

- 1 pound chicken breast, cut into bite-sized pieces
- 1 cup gluten-free flour mixture (such as rice flour or a gluten-free baking mix)
- 1 teaspoon garlic powder
- 1 teaspoon paprika
- 1/2 teaspoon salt

- 2 eggs, beaten

- 1 cup gluten-free breadcrumbs (or crushed gluten-free crackers)

- Cooking spray

Instructions:

1. Put parchment paper on a baking pan and preheat the oven to 400°F (200°C).

2. Combine the salt, paprika, garlic powder, and gluten-free flour in a bowl.

3. Beat the eggs in an other bowl.

4. The gluten-free breadcrumbs should be put in a third bowl.
5. Shake off any excess flour before dipping each piece of chicken into the sauce.

6. After that, coat the chicken with beaten eggs and then gluten-free breadcrumbs.

7. Place the coated chicken pieces on the baking sheet that has been prepared.

8. Apply cooking spray sparingly to the chicken nuggets.

9. Cook thoroughly and golden brown in the oven for 20 to 25 minutes.

10. Serve hot with the gluten-free dipping sauce of your child's choice.

Lettuce wraps with turkey

Ingredients:

- Sliced turkey breast, 1 pound
- 1 sliced avocado
- 8–10 large lettuce leaves, plus 1 large tomato, chopped
- To taste, add salt and pepper.

Instructions:

1. Lay out the lettuce leaves on a plate or cutting board.

2. Top each lettuce leaf with a few slices of turkey breast.

3. Add slices of avocado and chopped tomato on top of the turkey.

4. Season with salt and pepper to taste.

5. Roll up the lettuce leaves like a burrito, tucking in the sides as you go.

6. Serve cold and enjoy!

Quinoa Salad

Ingredients:

- 1 cup quinoa, rinsed
- 2 cups water or vegetable broth
- 1 red bell pepper, diced
- 1 cucumber, diced
- 1/2 red onion, diced

- 1/2 cup chopped fresh parsley

- 1/2 cup crumbled feta cheese (optional)

- 1/4 cup olive oil
- 3 tablespoons lemon juice

- 1 tablespoon honey

- 1/2 teaspoon ground cumin

- Salt and pepper, to taste

Instructions:

1. Bring the quinoa and water or broth to a boil in a medium pot.

2. When the quinoa is soft and the liquid has been absorbed, reduce the heat to low, cover the pan, and simmer for 15 to 20 minutes.

3. Quinoa should cool after the pot has been taken off the heat.

4. Combine the cooled quinoa with the diced red bell pepper, diced cucumber, diced red onion, and chopped parsley in a sizable bowl.

5. To create the dressing, combine the olive oil, lemon juice, honey, cumin, salt, and pepper in a separate small bowl.

6. Toss the quinoa salad with the dressing after adding it.
7. If preferred, top the salad with crumbled feta cheese.

8. Enjoy! Serve chilled or at room temperature.

Grilled Cheese Sandwich on Gluten-Free Bread

Ingredients:

- 2 slices gluten-free bread
- 2 slices cheddar cheese
- 1 tablespoon butter or margarine

Instructions:

1. Medium heat should be used to pre-heat a nonstick skillet.

2. Each piece of bread should be butter-side up.

3. In the skillet, put one slice of bread butter side down.

4. the bread in the skillet with the two slices of cheese on top.

5. The butter-side up should be facing the cheese when you place the second slice of bread on top.

6. Cook the bread for two to three minutes on each side, or until it is golden brown and the cheese is melted.

7. Enjoy when it's still hot!

Tuna Salad

Ingredients:

- 2 cans of tuna, drained

- 1/2 cup gluten-free mayonnaise
- 1/4 cup diced celery
- 1/4 cup diced red onion
- 1 tablespoon lemon juice
- Salt and pepper, to taste

Instructions:

1. Combine the tuna that has been drained, gluten-free mayonnaise, diced celery, diced red onion, and lemon juice in a big bowl.

2. Salt and pepper to taste should be added after a thorough mixing.

3. the flavors to mingle by chilling in the refrigerator for at least 30 minutes.

4. Enjoy! Spread this dish on gluten-free bread or crackers.

Gluten-Free Pizza

Ingredients:

- 1 gluten-free pizza crust
- 1/2 cup gluten-free tomato sauce
- 1 cup shredded mozzarella cheese
- Your child's favorite pizza toppings (such as sliced pepperoni, diced bell pepper, sliced mushrooms, or sliced olives)

Instructions:

1. The oven should be preheated at 425 degrees Fahrenheit.

2. The gluten-free pizza crust should be put on a baking pan.

3. Leaving a 1/2-inch margin around the edges, evenly spread the tomato sauce over the pizza crust.

4. Over the tomato sauce, top with shredded mozzarella cheese.

5. Pizza toppings of your child's choice should be added.

6. Until the cheese is melted and bubbling and the crust is golden brown, bake the pizza for 10 to 12 minutes.

7. Pizza should be taken out of the oven and allowed to cool before cutting.
8. Enjoy a hot serving!

Roasted Vegetable Salad

Ingredients:

- 2 cups mixed vegetables (such as cherry tomatoes, bell peppers, zucchini, and onion), chopped

- 1 tablespoon olive oil

- Salt and pepper, to taste

- 2 cups mixed greens

- Gluten-free dressing of your choice

Instructions:

1. Set the oven's temperature to 400 °F.

2. oil, salt, and pepper are added to the chopped vegetables.

3. On a baking sheet, distribute the vegetables in one layer.
4. For 20 to 25 minutes, or until soft and golden brown, roast the vegetables in the oven.
5. Toss the mixed greens in a sizable bowl with your preferred gluten-free dressing.

6. Toss the bowl with the added roasted vegetables.

7. Don't wait to serve; savor it!

Gluten-Free Mac and Cheese

Ingredients:

- 1 pound gluten-free elbow macaroni

- 1/4 cup butter or margarine

- 1/4 cup gluten-free flour

- 2 cups milk

- 2 cups shredded cheddar cheese

- Salt and pepper, to taste

Instructions:

1. As directed on the packaging, prepare the gluten-free elbow macaroni.

2. Butter should be melted over medium heat in a different pan.

3. Making a roux involves whisking in the gluten-free flour.

4. When the mixture is smooth, add the milk gradually while whisking continually.

5. For two to three minutes, or until thickened, bring the mixture to a simmer.

6. Cheddar cheese that has been shreddded should be added to the sauce.

7. With salt and pepper to taste, season the cheese sauce.

8. To the cheese sauce, add the cooked macaroni after draining.

9. Serve heated after stirring to mix.

Turkey and Avocado Wrap

Ingredients:

- 1 gluten-free tortilla
- 2 tablespoons mashed avocado
- 2 slices turkey
- 1/4 cup shredded lettuce

Instructions:

1. On the wheat-free tortilla, spread the mashed avocado.

2. On top of the avocado, arrange the sliced turkey.

3. Over the turkey, scatter the lettuce shreds.

4. To make a wrap, tightly roll the tortilla.

5. Serve the wrap by cutting it in half.

Grilled Salmon Skewers

Ingredients:

- 1 pound salmon fillets, cut into cubes
- 1/4 cup gluten-free soy sauce
- 1 tablespoon honey
- 2 cloves garlic, minced
- 1 tablespoon grated ginger
- 2 tablespoons olive oil

- Salt and pepper, to taste

- Skewers

Instructions:

1. To make the marinade, combine the honey, garlic, ginger, olive oil, salt, and pepper in a mixing bowl. The marinade should be gluten-free soy sauce.

2. Toss to coat the salmon cubes after adding them to the marinade.

3. Refrigerate for at least 30 minutes with a plastic wrap cover over the bowl.

4. Spend 10 to 15 minutes soaking the skewers in water.

5. Onto the skewers, thread the salmon cubes.

6. Medium-high heat should be applied to the grill.

7. Salmon skewers should be cooked all the way through on the grill for 3 to 4 minutes on each side.

8. Don't wait to serve; savor it!

Vegetable Stir-Fry

Ingredients:

- 2 cups mixed vegetables (such as bell peppers, onions, broccoli, and carrots), chopped

- 2 tablespoons olive oil

- 2 cloves garlic, minced

- 1 tablespoon grated ginger

- 2 tablespoons gluten-free soy sauce

- 1 tablespoon honey

- Salt and pepper, to taste

- Cooked rice, for serving

Instructions:

1. In a large skillet over medium-high heat, warm the olive oil.

2. Add the chopped vegetables and stir-fry for 3–4 minutes, or until crisp-tender.

3. Stir-fry the grated ginger and minced garlic in the skillet for 1–2 minutes, or until fragrant.

4. To make the sauce, combine the honey, salt, pepper, gluten-free soy sauce, and oil in a mixing bowl.

5. When the vegetables are thoroughly covered and the sauce is heated through, add the sauce to the skillet and stir-fry for 1-2 minutes.

6. Enjoy the veggie stir-fry over hot rice!

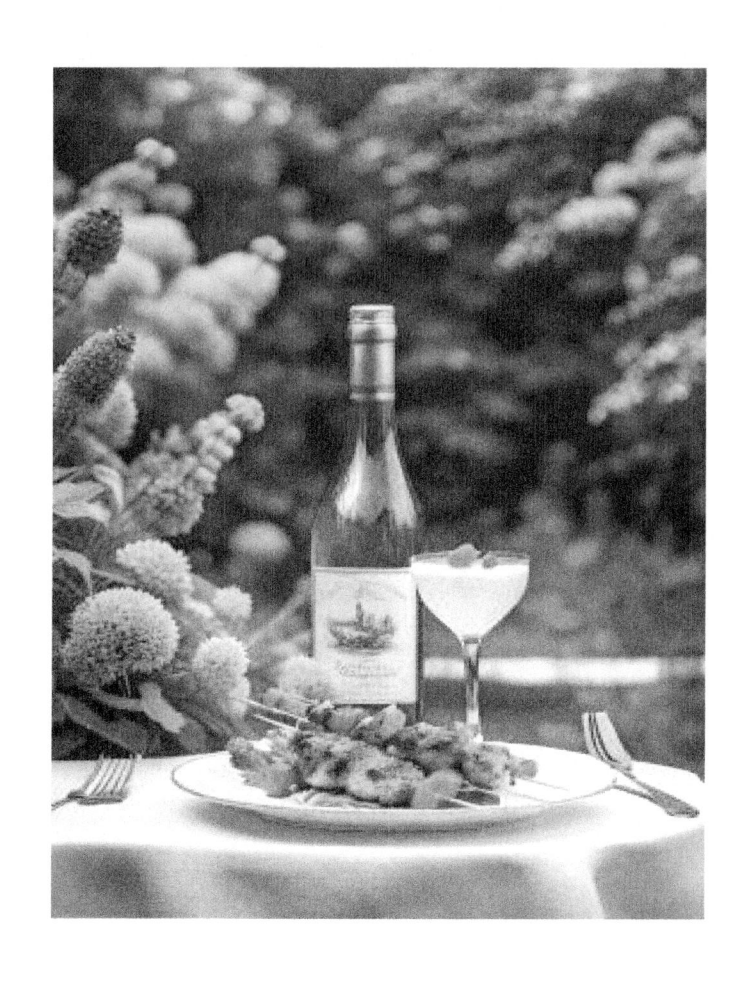

CHAPTER 4

DINNER RECIPE

This amazing dinner recipe, which is both gluten-free and overflowing with flavor, will blow your taste buds away. This recipe is ideal for children with celiac disease since it not only meets their nutritional needs but also makes them hanker after more. Every taste is certain to fascinate and delight thanks to the enticing combination of spices and ingredients. So let's begin this incredible gastronomic journey and explore the magical flavors that lie ahead.

Baked Chicken Tenders with Sweet Potato Fries

Ingredients:

- 1 pound chicken breast tenderloins
- 1 cup gluten-free bread crumbs
- 1 teaspoon paprika
- 1 teaspoon garlic powder

- Salt and pepper to taste

- 2 tablespoons olive oil

- 2 medium sweet potatoes, peeled and cut into fries

- 1 tablespoon cornstarch

- 1 tablespoon olive oil

- Salt and pepper to taste

Instructions:

1. Set the oven's temperature to 400°F (200°C).

2. Combine the bread crumbs, paprika, garlic powder, salt, and pepper in a small bowl.

3. Each chicken tenderloin is well coated after being dipped in the bread crumbs mixture.

4. Put the chicken tenders on a parchment paper-lined baking sheet.

5. tablespoons of olive oil should be drizzled over the chicken tenders.

6. On a different baking sheet that has been lined with parchment paper, arrange the sweet potato fries.

7. Combine the cornstarch, olive oil, salt, and pepper in a small bowl.

8. The sweet potato fries should be evenly coated after being tossed in the cornstarch mixture.

9. The chicken should be cooked through and the sweet potato fries should be crispy after 20 to 25 minutes in the preheated oven.

Gluten-free Pizza with a Cauliflower Crust and Toppings of Choice

Ingredients:

- 1 head cauliflower

- 1/2 cup gluten-free flour

- 1/2 cup grated parmesan cheese

- 1/2 teaspoon garlic powder

- 1/2 teaspoon dried basil

- 1/2 teaspoon dried oregano

- Salt and pepper to taste

- 1 egg, beaten

- 1/2 cup tomato sauce

- Toppings of your choice (such as shredded mozzarella cheese, pepperoni, sliced vegetables, etc.)

Instructions:

1. Set the oven's temperature to 400 °F (200 °C).

2. Cauliflower should be divided into florets, which should then be processed in a food processor until they resemble rice.

3. The cauliflower rice should be placed in a big bowl and heated in the microwave for 5-8 minutes, or until it is cooked through and soft.

4. The cauliflower should be transferred to a clean kitchen towel and wrung out as much moisture as you can after cooling for a few minutes.

5. Add the gluten-free flour, parmesan cheese, dried basil, dried oregano, salt, and pepper to the large bowl with the cauliflower after you've removed it. Blend thoroughly.

6. When you've thoroughly blended everything, add the beaten egg to the cauliflower mixture.

7. On a baking sheet covered with parchment paper, spread the cauliflower mixture and form it into a pizza crust shape.

8. Until the crust is golden brown, bake it in the preheated oven for 20 to 25 minutes.

9. Toppings of your choice should be added after the crust has been taken out of the oven.

10. When the cheese is melted and bubbling, put the pizza back in the oven for an additional 10 to 12 minutes of baking.

Grilled Salmon with Quinoa and Roasted Vegetables

Ingredients:

- 4 salmon fillets
- Salt and pepper to taste
- 2 tablespoons olive oil
- 1 cup quinoa
- 2 cups water or chicken broth
- 2 cups mixed vegetables (such as broccoli, bell peppers, zucchini, and onions), cut into bite-sized pieces
- 2 tablespoons olive oil
- Salt and pepper to taste

Instructions:

1. Set the grill's temperature to medium-high.
2. Two teaspoons of olive oil, salt, and pepper are used to season the salmon fillets.

3. The salmon fillets should be cooked through after grilling for 4–6 minutes on each side.

4. Rinse the quinoa, then add it to a medium pot with 2 cups of water or chicken stock as the salmon cooks.

5. When the liquid has been absorbed and the quinoa is tender, simmer the quinoa for 15 to 20 minutes after bringing it to a boil.

6. Set the oven's temperature to 400°F (200°C).

7. Place the mixed vegetables in a single layer on a baking sheet covered with parchment paper.

8. Add two tablespoons of olive oil to the veggies and season with salt and pepper to taste.

9. The veggies should be roasted for 20 to 25 minutes in a preheated oven, or until they are soft and gently browned.

10. Serve the grilled salmon with roasted veggies and a side of boiled quinoa.

Tacos made with Corn Tortillas, Ground Beef, and Avocado

Ingredients:

- 1 pound ground beef
- 1 tablespoon chili powder
- 1 teaspoon cumin
- Salt and pepper to taste
- 8 corn tortillas
- 1 avocado, sliced
- 1 cup shredded lettuce
- 1/2 cup shredded cheddar cheese
- Salsa and sour cream for serving (optional)

Turkey and Mashed Sweet Potatoes

Ingredients:

- 2 pounds sweet potatoes, peeled and chopped
- 1/4 cup milk or cream
- 2 tablespoons butter
- Salt and pepper to taste
- 1 pound ground turkey
- 1 onion, chopped
- 2 cloves garlic, minced
- 1 cup frozen peas and carrots
- 1 tablespoon tomato paste
- 1 tablespoon Worcestershire sauce
- 1 cup chicken or vegetable broth
- 1 tablespoon cornstarch

Instructions:

1. The oven should be heated to 375°F (190°C).

2. In a big saucepan of salted water, cook the sweet potatoes for 15 to 20 minutes, or until they are soft.

3. Sweet potatoes that have been drained should be mashed with butter, milk or cream, salt, and pepper to taste.

4. Until it is cooked through and browned, saute the ground turkey in a big skillet over medium heat.

5. The skillet should now contain the chopped onion and garlic. Cook for 2–3 minutes, or until the onion is transparent.

6. The tomato paste, Worcestershire sauce, and chicken or vegetable broth should all be stirred in after adding the frozen peas and carrots.

7. Put the cornstarch and 1 tablespoon of cold water in a small bowl and whisk to combine.

8. Stirring will be necessary after adding the cornstarch mixture to the skillet

9. Until the sauce has thickened, bring the mixture to a simmer and boil it for 5-7 minutes.

10. A 9x13-inch baking dish should be filled with the turkey mixture.

11. Spread the mashed sweet potatoes equally with a spatula and then add them on top of the turkey mixture.

12. The sweet potato topping should be gently browned and the filling bubbling, which should take 25 to 30 minutes in the preheated oven.

13. The Shepherd's Pie should cool down before being served. Enjoy!

Baked Ziti made with gluten-free pasta and ground beef or turkey

Ingredients:

- 1 pound gluten-free ziti or penne pasta
- 1 pound ground beef or turkey
- 1 onion, chopped
- 3 cloves garlic, minced

- 1 teaspoon dried oregano
- 1/2 teaspoon dried basil
- 1/4 teaspoon red pepper flakes
- Salt and pepper to taste
- 1 jar (24 ounces) gluten-free marinara sauce
- 2 cups shredded mozzarella cheese
- 1/4 cup grated Parmesan cheese

Instructions:

1. Set the oven to 375 degrees Fahrenheit (190 degrees Celsius).
2. According to the instructions on the package, prepare the gluten-free pasta until it is al dente.
3. The ground beef or turkey should be cooked thoroughly and browned in a sizable skillet over medium heat.

4. Cook the chopped onion and garlic in the skillet for two to three minutes, or until the onion is transparent.

5. Add the dried oregano, dry basil, red pepper flakes, salt, and pepper after stirring.

6. Stirring is required after adding the marinara sauce to the skillet.

7. Toss the cooked pasta with the sauce in the skillet after adding it.

8. A 9 x 13 inch baking dish should be filled with half of the spaghetti mixture.

9. The spaghetti mixture should be covered with 1 cup of the shredded mozzarella cheese.

10. Then, top with the remaining 1 cup of shredded mozzarella cheese and the grated Parmesan cheese. Add the leftover spaghetti mixture to the baking dish.

11. For 25 to 30 minutes, or until the cheese is melted and bubbling, bake the baked ziti in the preheated oven.

12. Prior to serving, let the baked ziti to cool for a short while. Enjoy!

Stuffed Bell Peppers with Ground Chicken and Quinoa

Ingredients:

- 4 bell peppers, tops removed and seeds removed
- 1 pound ground chicken
- 1 onion, chopped
- 2 cloves garlic, minced
- 1 cup cooked quinoa
- 1/2 cup gluten-free bread crumbs
- 1 egg, lightly beaten
- 1 teaspoon dried oregano
- Salt and pepper to taste
- 1 jar (24 ounces) gluten-free marinara sauce

Instructions:

1. The oven should be heated to 375°F (190°C).

2. Until it is cooked through and browned, sauté the ground chicken in a big skillet over medium heat.

3. The skillet should now contain the chopped onion and garlic. Cook for 2–3 minutes, or until the onion is transparent.

4. Cooked quinoa, egg, dried oregano, salt, and pepper, as well as gluten-free bread crumbs, should all be combined.

5. Stirring will help the sauce mix after being added to the skillet.

6. Pack the chicken and quinoa mixture tightly inside each bell pepper.

7. Put the stuffed bell peppers in a baking dish.

8. Over the stuffed bell peppers, add the leftover marinara sauce.

9. Bake the baking dish in the preheated oven for 45 to 50 minutes, or until the peppers are soft and the mixture is hot, with the foil covering it.

10. Before serving, let the stuffed bell peppers cool for a short while. Enjoy!

Grilled Chicken Skewers with Vegetables and Rice

Ingredients:

- 1 pound boneless, skinless chicken breast, cut into cubes

- 1 red bell pepper, cut into chunks

- 1 green bell pepper, cut into chunks

- 1 yellow onion, cut into chunks

- 8-10 wooden skewers, soaked in water for 30 minutes

- Salt and pepper to taste

- 2 tablespoons olive oil

- 2 cups cooked rice

Instructions:

1. Set the grill's temperature to medium-high.

2. Alternating between the ingredients, thread the skewers with the chicken, bell peppers, and onion.

3. Olive oil and salt and pepper should be used to season the skewers.

4. The skewers should be cooked through and slightly browned after 10 to 12 minutes of grilling, rotating them once or twice.

5. Cooked rice should be served alongside the skewers. Enjoy!

Beef Stir-Fry with Broccoli and Gluten-Free Tamari Sauce

Ingredients:

- 1 pound flank steak, sliced thinly against the grain
- 3 tablespoons gluten-free tamari sauce
- 2 tablespoons honey
- 1 tablespoon cornstarch
- 1 tablespoon sesame oil
- 3 cloves garlic, minced
- 1 tablespoon grated fresh ginger
- 1 head broccoli, cut into florets
- 1 red bell pepper, sliced
- Salt and pepper to taste
- Cooked rice, for serving

Instructions:

1. Mix the gluten-free tamari sauce, honey, cornstarch, and 1/4 cup water in a small bowl until combined and smooth.

2. Sesame oil should be heated to a high temperature in a big skillet or wok.

3. In the skillet, add the flank steak slices and cook for 2 to 3 minutes, or until browned all over. Take the steak out of the skillet and place it aside.

4. Cook the grated ginger and minced garlic in the skillet for one to two minutes, or until fragrant.

5. When the vegetables are tender-crisp, add the broccoli and bell pepper slices to the skillet. Cook the vegetables for 3–4 minutes.

6. The tamari sauce mixture should be poured over the vegetables, then combined.

7. After the vegetables and sauce have been added, add the cooked flank steak back to the skillet.

8. Cook the steak for a further one to two minutes, or until it is well heated and the sauce has thickened.

9. Serve cooked rice alongside the meat stir-fry. Enjoy!

Chicken Parmesan made with Gluten-Free Bread Crumbs

Ingredients:

- 4 boneless, skinless chicken breasts
- 1 cup gluten-free bread crumbs
- 1/2 cup grated Parmesan cheese
- 2 teaspoons Italian seasoning
- Salt and pepper to taste
- 2 eggs, beaten
- 1/4 cup olive oil
- 1 jar (24 ounces) gluten-free marinara sauce
- 1 cup shredded mozzarella cheese

Instructions:

1. Set the oven to 375 degrees Fahrenheit.

2. Blend the Italian seasoning, grated Parmesan cheese, salt, and pepper with the gluten-free bread crumbs in a shallow dish.

3. Before being covered in the bread crumbs, each chicken breast is first dipped in the beaten eggs.

4. Olive oil should be heated to a medium-high temperature in a big skillet. Add the chicken breasts and cook for 3–4 minutes until golden brown on each side.

5. Then, add marinara sauce and shredded mozzarella cheese to the top of each chicken breast before placing the chicken in a baking dish.

6. Cook the chicken in the oven for 25 to 30 minutes, or until the cheese is melted and bubbling.

7. A side of gluten-free pasta or veggies should be served with the chicken parmesan, along with more marinara sauce. Enjoy!

Cauliflower Fried Rice with Shrimp or Chicken
Ingredients:

- 1 head cauliflower, grated
- 1 pound shrimp or chicken, peeled and deveined
- 1 cup frozen peas and carrots
- 1/2 cup diced onion
- 2 cloves garlic, minced
- 1 tablespoon coconut oil
- 2 eggs, beaten
- 3 tablespoons gluten-free tamari sauce
- 2 tablespoons chopped green onions
- Salt and pepper to taste

Instructions:

1. The coconut oil should be heated over medium-high heat in a sizable skillet or wok.

2. Cook the minced garlic and diced onion in the skillet for two to three minutes until fragrant.

3. The chicken or shrimp should be added to the skillet and cooked thoroughly after 5–6 minutes.

4. Once the frozen peas and carrots have thawed and heated thoroughly, add them to the skillet.

5. Add the beaten eggs to the empty area left by moving the skillet's contents to the side. The eggs should be boiled through before being scrambled and combined with the remaining ingredients.

6. Grated cauliflower should be added to the skillet and mixed with the remaining ingredients.

7. To uniformly coat the cauliflower mixture, drizzle the tamari sauce over it and toss.

8. Cook the cauliflower for 3 to 4 minutes, or until it is heated through and is tender-crisp.

9. Before serving, season to taste with salt and pepper and sprinkle with finely sliced green onions. Enjoy!

Slow Cooker Chicken and Vegetable Soup with Gluten-Free Noodles

Ingredients:

- 1 pound boneless, skinless chicken breasts, diced
- 6 cups gluten-free chicken broth
- 2 cups diced carrots
- 2 cups diced celery
- 1 cup diced onion
- 3 cloves garlic, minced
- 1 teaspoon dried thyme
- 1 teaspoon dried rosemary
- Salt and pepper to taste
- 8 ounces gluten-free noodles (such as rice noodles or quinoa noodles)

Instructions:

1. Put the diced chicken, chicken broth, carrots, celery, onion, garlic, thyme, rosemary, salt, and pepper in a slow cooker.

2. When the chicken is cooked through and the vegetables are soft, cook on high for 3–4 hours or on low for 6–8 hours.

3. Add the gluten-free noodles and mix them into the slow cooker during the last 20 to 30 minutes of cooking.

4. Serve the soup hot after continuing to cook the soup until the noodles are ready. Enjoy!

Baked Salmon Cakes with Roasted Sweet Potato Wedges

Ingredients:

- 1 pound salmon fillet, skin removed
- 1/4 cup gluten-free bread crumbs
- 1/4 cup finely chopped red onion
- 2 tablespoons chopped fresh parsley
- 1 egg, beaten
- Salt and pepper to taste

- 2 large sweet potatoes, cut into wedges
- 2 tablespoons olive oil
- 1 teaspoon garlic powder
- 1 teaspoon paprika

Instructions:

1. Set the oven to 375 degrees Fahrenheit.

2. Fork-flake the fish into small pieces and place in a big bowl.

3. In the bowl containing the salmon, mix the egg, salt, pepper, red onion, gluten-free bread crumbs, parsley, and red onion. In a large bowl, thoroughly combine all the ingredients.

4. Form each portion of the mixture into a patty by dividing it into 8 equal portions.

5. Placing the salmon patties on a baking pan with parchment paper can help prevent sticking.

6. Olive oil, paprika, garlic powder, salt, and pepper should all be combined in a different bowl.
7. The sweet potato wedges should be evenly coated after being tossed in the oil mixture.

8. Place the salmon patties and sweet potato wedges on the baking sheet.

9. Bake the salmon for 20 to 25 minutes, or until it is done, and the sweet potatoes are soft and browned.

10. Along with the roasted sweet potato wedges and your preferred gluten-free dipping sauce, serve the salmon cakes. Enjoy!

Sloppy Joes made with Gluten-Free Buns and Ground Turkey or Beef

Ingredients:

- 1 pound ground turkey or beef

- 1 tablespoon olive oil

- 1 cup diced onion

- 1 cup diced green bell pepper
- 2 cloves garlic, minced
- 1 cup gluten-free tomato sauce
- 1/4 cup gluten-free ketchup
- 2 tablespoons gluten-free Worcestershire sauce
- 2 tablespoons brown sugar
- Salt and pepper to taste
- Gluten-free buns for serving

Instructions:

1. In a large skillet over medium-high heat, warm the olive oil.

2. Garlic, onion, green bell pepper, and ground beef or turkey should all be added to the skillet. Cook, occasionally stirring, until the meat is browned and the vegetables are soft.

3. Remove any extra grease from the skillet.

4. Add the tomato sauce, ketchup, Worcestershire sauce, brown sugar, salt, and pepper. Turn the heat down to low and simmer the mixture for 10 to 15 minutes, or until the flavors are well-balanced and the sauce has thickened.

5. Serve the sloppy joe mixture on buns free of gluten. Enjoy!

Vegetable and Quinoa Stuffed Portobello Mushrooms

Ingredients:

- 4 large portobello mushrooms, stems removed
- 1 cup cooked quinoa
- 1 cup diced zucchini
- 1 cup diced red bell pepper
- 1/2 cup diced onion
- 2 cloves garlic, minced
- 1/4 cup chopped fresh parsley

- 1/4 cup grated Parmesan cheese

- Salt and pepper to taste

- 2 tablespoons olive oil

Instructions:

1. Set the oven to 375 degrees Fahrenheit.

2. Put the cooked quinoa, zucchini, red bell pepper, onion, garlic, parsley, Parmesan cheese, salt, and pepper in a sizable bowl.

3. The quinoa and vegetable mixture should be placed inside each portobello mushroom cap using a spoon, packing it in carefully.

4. Olive oil should be drizzled over each mushroom.

5. On a baking sheet covered with parchment paper, put the stuffed mushrooms.

6. Bake for 20 to 25 minutes, or until the mushrooms are cooked through and the filling is thoroughly warmed.

7. With more chopped parsley as a garnish, if desired, serve the packed mushrooms hot. Enjoy!

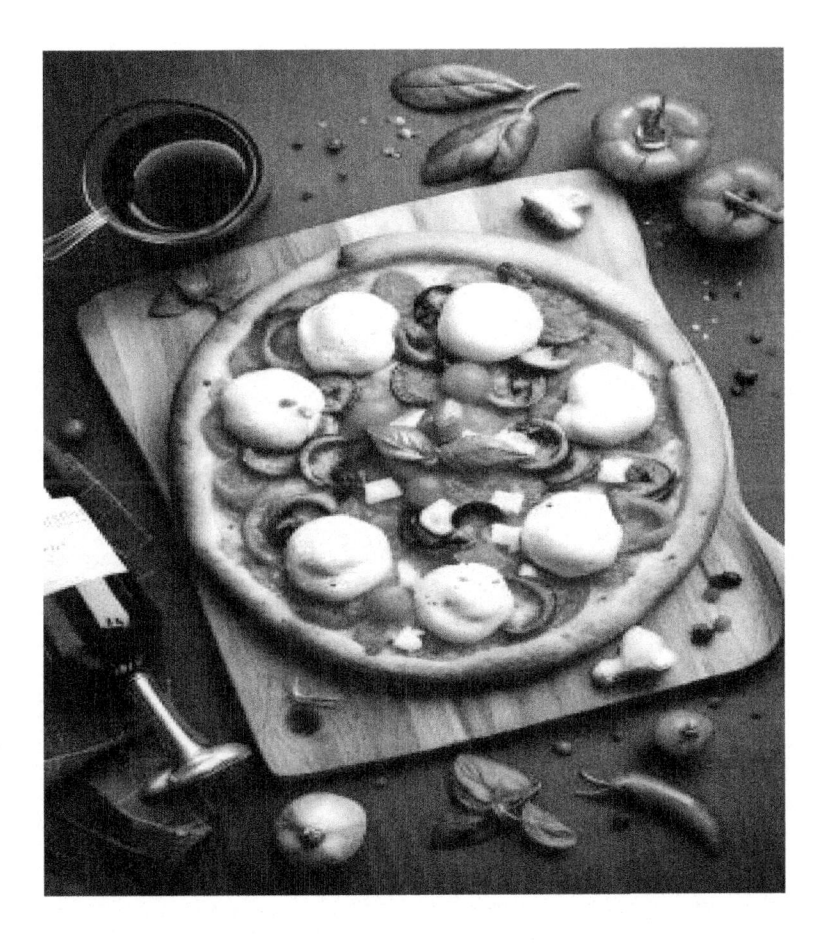

CHAPTER 5

SNACK AND SIDE DISH RECIPES

Every meal should include snacks and side dishes since they bring taste and additional nutrients. To guarantee that children with Celiac disease are not consuming any gluten, it is crucial to choose gluten-free products. Here are some recipes for snacks and sides:

Baked Sweet Potato Fries

Ingredients:

- 2 medium sweet potatoes
- 2 tablespoons olive oil
- 1 teaspoon paprika
- 1 teaspoon garlic powder
- 1/2 teaspoon salt

Instructions:

1. Set your oven's temperature to 400°F (200°C).

2. Cut the sweet potatoes into 1/4-inch-thick fries.

3. Olive oil, paprika, garlic powder, and salt should all be combined in a basin.

4. Once the sweet potato fries are added, mix them in the bowl so that the oil and seasonings are distributed equally.

5. Put the fries on a baking sheet that has been covered with parchment paper in a single layer.

6. Bake the fries until they are crispy and golden brown for 20 to 25 minutes, flipping them halfway through.

7. Enjoy a hot serving!

Roasted Chickpeas

Ingredients:

- 1 can chickpeas (15 oz.), drained and rinsed
- 1 tablespoon olive oil
- 1/2 teaspoon smoked paprika
- 1/2 teaspoon cumin
- 1/2 teaspoon garlic powder
- 1/4 teaspoon salt

Instructions:

1. Set your oven's temperature to 400°F (200°C).
2. Utilizing a paper towel, pat the chickpeas dry.
3. Salt, cumin, smoked paprika, garlic powder, and olive oil should all be combined in a bowl.
4. Add the chickpeas and stir until they are equally covered in the oil and seasonings.
5. On a parchment paper-lined baking sheet, spread the chickpeas out in a single layer.

6. Bake the chickpeas until crispy and golden brown for 20 to 25 minutes, shaking the baking sheet every so often.

7. Serve warm or at room temperature and take pleasure!

Cucumber and Tomato Salad

Ingredients:

- 1 large cucumber, sliced //
- 1 pint cherry tomatoes, halved
- 1/4 cup crumbled feta cheese
- 2 tablespoons olive oil
- 1 tablespoon fresh lemon juice
- 1 tablespoon chopped fresh parsley
- Salt and pepper, to taste

Instructions:

1. Combine the cucumber, cherry tomatoes, and feta cheese in a bowl.

2. Combine the parsley, olive oil, lemon juice, salt, and pepper in a separate bowl.

3. After adding the dressing, toss the cucumber and tomato mixture to evenly distribute the dressing.

4. Before serving, place in the refrigerator for at least 10 minutes to enable the flavors to mingle.

5. Enjoy a chilled serving!

Guacamole

Ingredients:

- 3 ripe avocados
- Juice of 1 lime
- 1/2 teaspoon salt
- 1/4 teaspoon cumin
- 1/4 teaspoon garlic powder

- 1/4 teaspoon onion powder

- 1/4 teaspoon cayenne pepper (optional)

- 2 tablespoons chopped fresh cilantro (optional)

Instructions:

1. Remove the pit from the avocados after cutting them in half. Place the flesh in a basin by scooping.

2. To the bowl, add the lime juice, salt, cumin, garlic powder, onion powder, and cayenne pepper (if using).

3. Use a fork or potato masher to mash the avocado mixture until it has the consistency you want.

4. Add the chopped cilantro, if using.

5. When necessary, taste and adjust the seasoning.

6. Serve with tortilla chips or vegetables and take pleasure in it!

Caprese Skewers

Ingredients:

- 1 pint cherry tomatoes
- 8 ounces fresh mozzarella, cut into bite-sized pieces
- Fresh basil leaves
- Balsamic glaze

Instructions:

1. A basil leaf, a piece of mozzarella, and a cherry tomato should all be skewered together.
2. Continue until every ingredient has been utilized.
3. Balsamic glaze should be applied to the skewers.
4. Enjoy! Serve chilled or at room temperature.

Hummus and Veggies

Ingredients:

- 1 cup store-bought or homemade hummus

- Sliced carrots

- Sliced celery

- Sliced bell peppers

Instructions:

1. Put the hummus in a bowl and set it aside.

2. The vegetables should be washed and cut into slices.

3. Place the vegetables close to the hummus bowl.

4. Serve and take pleasure!

Popcorn with Nutritional Yeast

Ingredients:

- 1/2 cup popcorn kernels

- 2 tablespoons nutritional yeast

- 2 tablespoons melted butter or olive oil

- Salt, to taste

Instructions:

1. In a big bowl, add the popped popcorn kernels after popping them in accordance with the directions on the package.

2. Pop the popcorn and toss to coat with the melted butter or olive oil.

3. When the popcorn is properly covered, sprinkle the salt and nutritional yeast over it.

4. Enjoy after serving!

Baked Buffalo Cauliflower Bites

Ingredients:

- 1 head cauliflower, cut into bite-sized pieces

- 1/2 cup buffalo sauce

- 1/2 cup breadcrumbs

- Salt and pepper, to taste

- Ranch dressing, for dipping (optional)

Instructions:

1. Put parchment paper on a baking pan and preheat the oven to 400°F (200°C).

2. Buffalo sauce and cauliflower pieces should be combined in a sizable bowl and mixed thoroughly.

3. Breadcrumbs, salt, and pepper should all be combined in a different bowl.

4. Each piece of cauliflower should be dipped into the breadcrumb mixture and coated carefully.

5. On the baking sheet that has been prepared, arrange the cauliflower pieces in a single layer.

6. Bake for 20 to 25 minutes, or until the breadcrumbs are golden and crispy and the cauliflower is soft.

7. Enjoy! Serve hot with ranch dressing on the side for dipping, if desired.

Deviled Eggs

Ingredients:

- 6 hard-boiled eggs, peeled and halved lengthwise
- 2 tablespoons mayonnaise
- 1 tablespoon Dijon mustard
- 1/2 teaspoon paprika
- Salt and pepper, to taste
- Chopped fresh chives, for garnish (optional)

Instructions:

1. The yolks from the eggs should be removed and put in a bowl.

2. The yolks should be crumbly after being thoroughly mashed with a fork.

3. In a bowl, combine the mayonnaise, mustard, paprika, salt, and pepper.

4. Return the yolk mixture to the egg whites and distribute it evenly.

5. If using, garnish with chopped chives.

6. Serve and take pleasure!

Spinach and Artichoke Dip

Ingredients:

- 1 (10 oz) package frozen chopped spinach, thawed and drained

- 1 (14 oz) can artichoke hearts, drained and chopped

- 8 oz cream cheese, softened

- 1/2 cup grated Parmesan cheese

- 1/4 cup mayonnaise

- 2 cloves garlic, minced

- Salt and pepper, to taste

Instructions:

1. Prepare a small baking dish with grease and preheat the oven to 375°F (190°C).

2. Mix the spinach, artichoke hearts, mayonnaise, cream cheese, Parmesan cheese, salt, and pepper in a sizable bowl.

3. Smooth the top of the mixture before transferring it to the prepared baking dish.

4. Bake the dip for 20 to 25 minutes, or until it is heated and bubbling.

5. Enjoy by serving with tortilla chips, pita chips, or vegetables for dipping.

Sweet and Spicy Mixed Nuts

Ingredients:

- 2 cups mixed nuts (such as almonds, cashews, and pecans)

- 2 tablespoons honey
- 1 tablespoon sriracha
- 1 teaspoon smoked paprika
- 1/2 teaspoon salt

Instructions:

1. A baking sheet should be lined with parchment paper and the oven should be preheated to 350°F (175°C).

2. Mix the nuts in a large bowl and toss with the honey, sriracha, smoked paprika, and salt to coat.

3. On the prepared baking sheet, arrange the nuts in a single layer.

4. Bake the nuts until they are aromatic and golden brown for 10 to 15 minutes, stirring once or twice.

5. Before serving, let the nuts cool fully. Have fun!

Pita Chips and Tzatziki

Ingredients:

- 4 pita breads
- 2 tablespoons olive oil
- 1/2 teaspoon garlic powder
- Salt and pepper, to taste
- 1 cup plain Greek yogurt
- 1/2 cup grated cucumber
- 1 clove garlic, minced
- 1 tablespoon lemon juice
- 1 tablespoon chopped fresh dill

Instructions:

1. Set a baking sheet on the counter and preheat the oven to 375°F (190°C).

2. On the pre-heated baking sheet, spread out each pita bread wedge into a single layer.

3. Olive oil, garlic powder, salt, and pepper should all be combined in a small basin.

4. After brushing the pita wedges with the oil mixture, bake for 10 to 12 minutes, or until crispy and golden brown.

5. Combine the grated cucumber, garlic, lemon juice, dill, and Greek yogurt in a separate bowl.

6. Tzatziki should be served alongside the pita chips for dipping.

Bruschetta

Ingredients:

- 1 baguette or Italian bread, sliced
- 3-4 ripe tomatoes, diced
- 2 cloves garlic, minced

- 2-3 tablespoons fresh basil, chopped

- 1 tablespoon balsamic glaze

- Salt and pepper, to taste

- Olive oil, for brushing

Instructions:

1. The oven should be heated to 375°F (190°C).

2. Brush olive oil on the bread slices and arrange them on a baking pan.

3. Toasted and golden brown bread should be baked for 10 to 12 minutes.

4. Combine the chopped tomatoes with the balsamic glaze, salt, pepper, garlic, and basil in a bowl.

5. Toasted bread pieces should be covered with the tomato mixture before serving.

Baked Zucchini Fries

Ingredients:

- 2 medium zucchini, cut into fries

- 1/2 cup breadcrumbs

- 1/2 cup grated Parmesan cheese
- 2 tablespoons olive oil

- 1/2 teaspoon garlic powder

- Salt and pepper, to taste

- Marinara sauce, for dipping

Instructions:

1. Set a baking sheet on the counter and preheat the oven to 425°F (220°C).

2. Breadcrumbs, Parmesan cheese, olive oil, garlic powder, salt, and pepper should all be combined in a big bowl.

3. Each zucchini fry should be dipped into the breadcrumb mixture and coated thoroughly by pressing the crumbs onto the zucchini.

4. Put a single layer of the coated zucchini fries on the baking sheet that has been prepared.

5. Bake the fries until they are golden brown and crispy for 20 to 25 minutes, flipping them halfway through.

6. Enjoy while dipping into marinara sauce!

Stuffed Mushrooms

Ingredients:

- 12-16 large mushrooms, stems removed
- 8 oz cream cheese, softened
- 2 cloves garlic, minced
- 2 tablespoons fresh herbs (such as parsley, thyme, or basil), chopped
- 1/2 cup grated Parmesan cheese
- Salt and pepper, to taste

Instructions:

1. Bake at 375°F (190°C) for 15 minutes with a baking sheet lined with parchment paper.

2. Mix the cream cheese, garlic, herbs, Parmesan cheese, salt, and pepper in a bowl until well combined.

3. Fill each mushroom cap completely with the cream cheese mixture before placing it there.

4. The stuffed mushrooms should be baked for 20 to 25 minutes, or until the filling is golden brown and the mushrooms are soft.

5. Serving hot, please.

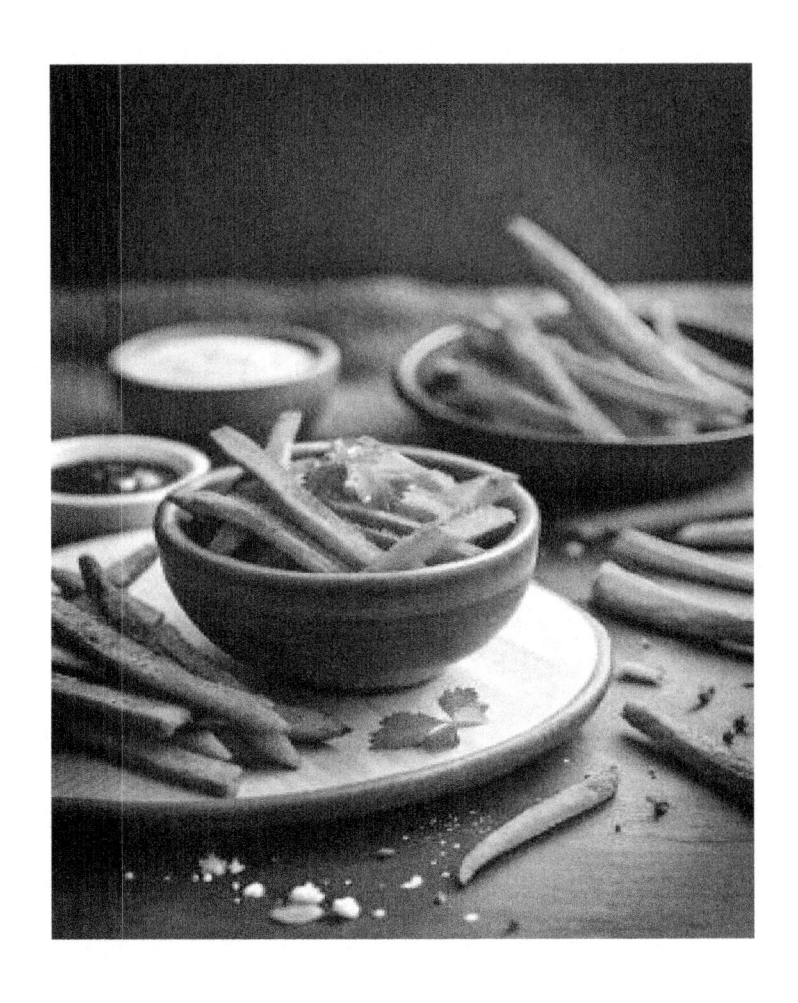

CHAPTER 6

DESSERT RECIPES

Desserts are a fun and delectable way to enjoy a sweet treat, but for children with Celiac disease, it's crucial to find gluten-free options to guarantee they aren't absorbing any gluten. Here are some delicious and gluten-free dessert dish ideas:

Classic Chocolate Chip Cookies

Ingredients:

- 2 1/4 cups all-purpose flour
- 1 tsp baking soda
- 1 tsp salt
- 1 cup unsalted butter, softened
- 3/4 cup granulated sugar
- 3/4 cup brown sugar, packed

- 2 large eggs

- 2 tsp vanilla extract

- 2 cups semisweet chocolate chips

Instructions:

1. Your oven should be preheated at 375°F (190°C).

2. Mix the salt, baking soda, and flour in a medium-sized bowl.

3. Butter, brown sugar, and granulated sugar are combined in a sizable mixing basin and creamed until frothy.

4. When thoroughly blended, add the eggs and vanilla extract.

5. Stirring until just mixed, gradually add the flour mixture.

6. Add the chocolate chips after stirring.

7. On a baking sheet with parchment paper already attached, drop spoonfuls of the dough.

8. To softly brown edges, bake for 8 to 10 minutes.

9. Prior to moving the cookies to a wire rack to finish cooling, let them cool on the baking sheet for a short while.

Fudgy Brownies

Ingredients:

- 1 cup unsalted butter
- 2 1/4 cups granulated sugar
- 1 1/4 cups unsweetened cocoa powder
- 1 tsp salt
- 1 tsp baking powder
- 1 tsp espresso powder
- 1 tbsp vanilla extract
- 4 large eggs
- 1 1/2 cups all-purpose flour

- 2 cups semisweet chocolate chips

Instructions:

1. Turn on the oven to 350 °F (175 °C).

2. Melt the butter in a sizable mixing basin using a microwave.

3. Until thoroughly blended, stir in the sugar, cocoa powder, salt, baking powder, espresso powder, and vanilla extract.

4. One at a time, beat in the eggs until thoroughly incorporated.

5. Stir in the flour a little at a time until barely mixed.

6. Add the chocolate chunks and stir.

7. In a 9x13-inch baking dish that has been lined with parchment paper, pour the batter.

8. Bake for 30-35 minutes, or until moist crumbs come out when a toothpick is inserted in the center.

9. Before cutting and serving, let the brownies cool completely in the baking dish.

Vanilla Bean Cupcakes with Buttercream Frosting

Ingredients:

(a.) For the cupcakes:

- 1 3/4 cups all-purpose flour
- 1 tsp baking powder
- 1/2 tsp baking soda
- 1/2 tsp salt
- 1/2 cup unsalted butter, softened
- 1 cup granulated sugar
- 2 large eggs
- 2 tsp vanilla bean paste
- 1 cup whole milk

(b.) For the buttercream frosting:

- 1 cup unsalted butter, softened
- 4 cups powdered sugar
- 1/4 cup heavy cream
- 2 tsp vanilla extract

Instructions:

1. Set your oven's temperature to 350 °F (175 °C).

2. Baking soda, salt, baking powder, and flour should be combined in a medium-sized bowl.

3. Butter and granulated sugar should be creamed until frothy in a large mixing bowl.

4. When thoroughly blended, add the eggs one at a time.

5. Stir in the vanilla bean paste.
6. Mixture should just come together after you gradually alternate adding milk and flour.

7. Each cupcake liner should be filled 2/3 of the way with the batter after lining a muffin pan.

8. When a toothpick put in the center of the cake comes out clean, bake for 18 to 20 minutes.

9. In order to properly frost the cupcakes, let them cool fully.

For the buttercream frosting:

1. Beat the butter in a sizable mixing basin until it is light and creamy.

2. Add the powdered sugar gradually, 1 cup at a time, until thoroughly blended.

3. The frosting will become smooth and creamy when you've added the heavy cream and vanilla extract.

4. When the cupcakes are cool, pipe on the icing and add any desired decorations.

Lemon Bars

Ingredients:

(a.) For the crust:

- 1 cup unsalted butter, softened
- 1/2 cup granulated sugar
- 2 cups all-purpose flour
- 1/4 tsp salt

(b.) For the filling:

- 4 large eggs
- 1 1/2 cups granulated sugar
- 1/2 cup fresh lemon juice
- 1/4 cup all-purpose flour
- 1/2 tsp baking powder
- 1/4 tsp salt
- Powdered sugar, for dusting

Instructions:

1. Set your oven's temperature to 350 °F (175 °C).

2. Butter and granulated sugar should be creamed until frothy in a large mixing bowl.

3. Once the mixture starts to resemble dough, add the flour and salt gradually.

4. Using parchment paper as a liner, press the dough into a 9x13-inch baking pan.

5. Until the edges are just beginning to turn golden, bake for 18 to 20 minutes.

6. By thoroughly combining the eggs, granulated sugar, lemon juice, flour, baking soda, and salt, you may make the filling while the crust is baking.

7. A further 18 to 20 minutes of baking, or until the filling is set, should be added after pouring the filling over the hot crust.

8. Toss the bars with powdered sugar and cut them into squares after they have totally cooled.

Cinnamon Rolls with Cream Cheese Frosting

Ingredients:

(a.) For the dough:

- 4 cups all-purpose flour
- 1/4 cup granulated sugar
- 2 1/4 tsp instant yeast
- 1 tsp salt
- 1/2 cup unsalted butter, softened
- 1/2 cup whole milk
- 1/4 cup water
- 2 large eggs

(b.) For the filling:

- 1/2 cup unsalted butter, softened
- 1/2 cup granulated sugar
- 1/4 cup brown sugar

- 2 tbsp ground cinnamon

(c.) For the cream cheese frosting:

- 4 oz cream cheese, softened
- 1/4 cup unsalted butter, softened
- 1 1/2 cups powdered sugar
- 1 tsp vanilla extract

Instructions:

1. Combine the flour, salt, yeast, and granulated sugar in a sizable mixing basin.

2. Butter, milk, and water should be heated in a small saucepan until the butter has melted and the liquid is warm to the touch.

3. The dry ingredients should be combined with the warm liquid mixture and eggs to produce a dough.

4. On a floured surface, knead the dough for 5 to 10 minutes, or until it is smooth and elastic.

5. The dough should be placed in an oiled basin, covered with a moist towel, and allowed to rise for an hour in a warm location.

6. Grease a 9x13-inch baking dish and preheat the oven to 375°F (190°C).

7. On a surface dusted with flour, roll out the dough into a broad rectangle.

8. The granulated sugar, brown sugar, and cinnamon are strewn over the dough once the softened butter has been spread over it.

9. The dough should be formed into a tight log that is then cut into 12 equal pieces.

10. The cinnamon rolls should be baked for 25 to 30 minutes, or until just softly golden brown, in the buttered baking dish.

11. Prepare the cream cheese frosting by beating the cream cheese, butter, icing sugar, and vanilla extract until creamy while the cinnamon rolls are baking.

12. After taking the cinnamon buns out of the oven, let them cool a little before covering them with cream cheese frosting.

Strawberry Shortcake

Ingredients:

(a.) For the shortcakes:

- 2 cups all-purpose flour

- 1/4 cup granulated sugar

- 1 tbsp baking powder

- 1/2 tsp salt

- 1/2 cup cold unsalted butter, cut into small pieces

- 2/3 cup cold heavy cream
- 1 large egg, lightly beaten

- Coarse sugar, for sprinkling

(b.) For the strawberries:

- 2 pounds fresh strawberries, hulled and sliced
- 1/4 cup granulated sugar
- For the whipped cream:
- 1 1/2 cups cold heavy cream
- 1/4 cup powdered sugar
- 1 tsp vanilla extract

Instructions:

1. Place a baking sheet in the oven and preheat it to 400°F (205°C).

2. The flour, brown sugar, baking soda, and salt should all be combined in a sizable mixing dish.

3. The cold butter should be incorporated using a pastry blender or your fingers until the mixture resembles coarse crumbs.

4. Stir in the heavy cream until the dough comes together after adding it.

5. To make the dough smooth, spread it out on a surface that has been lightly dusted with flour.

6. Using a biscuit cutter or a round cookie cutter, cut out 6 to 8 shortcakes from the rolled-out dough at a thickness of 1/2 inch.

7. Shortcakes should be placed onto the baking sheet that has been preheated, then they should be brushed with a gently beaten egg and dusted with coarse sugar.

8. To achieve golden brown results, bake for 15 to 18 minutes.

9. Put the strawberries in a medium bowl with the sugar and prepare the shortcakes while they bake.

10. While you make the whipped cream, set aside the strawberry mixture to macerate.

11. Cold heavy cream, powdered sugar, and vanilla extract should be combined and beaten until stiff peaks form in a large mixing basin.

12. Cut the cooled shortcakes horizontally in half to assemble the strawberry shortcakes.

13. Add a dollop of whipped cream and a few of the macerated strawberries to the bottom of each shortcake.

14. Add the second half of the shortcake on top, then serve right away. Enjoy!

Blueberry Crisp

Ingredients:

- 4 cups fresh blueberries
- 1/2 cup all-purpose flour
- 1/2 cup rolled oats
- 1/2 cup brown sugar
- 1/2 tsp ground cinnamon
- 1/4 tsp salt
- 1/2 cup unsalted butter, chilled and cubed

Instructions:

1. Pre-heat your oven to 375°F (190°C), then butter a 9-inch baking dish.

2. Spread the blueberries evenly in the prepared baking dish after tossing them in a sizable mixing basin with 1/4 cup of the flour.

3. The remaining 1/4 cup of flour, rolled oats, brown sugar, ground cinnamon, and salt should be combined with the other ingredients in a separate mixing dish.

4. When the flour mixture resembles coarse crumbs, add the cold, cubed butter to the bowl and blend it in with a pastry cutter or your fingers.

5. The blueberries in the baking dish will have the topping sprinkled over them.

6. For 35 to 40 minutes, or until the topping is golden brown and the blueberries are bubbling, bake the blueberry crisp.
7. If ice cream is preferred, top the heated dish with a scoop before serving.

Chocolate Mousse

Ingredients:

- 8 oz semi-sweet chocolate, chopped
- 4 large eggs, separated
- 1/4 cup granulated sugar
- 1/4 cup unsalted butter, softened
- 1/4 cup heavy cream
- 1/2 tsp vanilla extract
- Pinch of salt

Instructions:

1. Using a double boiler or a microwave, melt the chopped chocolate until it is smooth. Allow it to gently cool.

2. The egg yolks and sugar should be combined in a sizable mixing basin and whisked until frothy.

3. Mix everything together in the basin after adding the softened butter.

4. Add the melted chocolate and continue beating until smooth.

5. The egg whites and a dash of salt should be beaten in another mixing basin until stiff peaks form.

6. Beat the heavy cream and vanilla extract in another bowl until soft peaks form.

7. Gently incorporate the whipped cream into the chocolate mixture after you've added the beaten egg whites.

8. When chilled for at least two hours or until solid, divide the chocolate mousse among 4-6 serving dishes.

9. If preferred, top off the cold dish with whipped cream and grated chocolate.

Apple Pie with Crumb Topping

Ingredients:

(a.) For the crust:

- 2 1/2 cups all-purpose flour
- 1 tsp salt
- 1 tbsp granulated sugar
- 1 cup unsalted butter, cold and cubed
- 1/4 to 1/2 cup ice water

(b.) For the filling:

- 6 cups peeled and thinly sliced apples
- 1/2 cup granulated sugar
- 1/4 cup brown sugar
- 1 tsp ground cinnamon
- 1/4 tsp ground nutmeg
- 1/4 tsp salt
- 3 tbsp all-purpose flour

(c.) For the crumb topping:

- 1/2 cup all-purpose flour

- 1/4 cup brown sugar

- 1/4 cup granulated sugar
- 1 tsp ground cinnamon

- 1/4 tsp salt

- 6 tbsp unsalted butter, cold and cubed

Instructions:

1. Prepare a 9-inch pie plate with oil and preheat the oven to 375°F (190°C).

2. For the crust, combine the flour, salt, and sugar in a sizable mixing basin.

3. Use a pastry cutter or your fingers to cut the cold, cubed butter into the flour mixture until it resembles coarse crumbs after adding it to the bowl.

4. One spoonful at a time, add the ice water to the bowl while stirring continuously until the dough comes together.

5. The dough should be divided in half, with one half being rolled out to fit the pie dish on a floured surface. Trim the borders, then put it in the pie dish.

6. Fill the pie crust with the apple mixture.

7. For the crumb topping, blend the flour, sugars, cinnamon, and salt in a separate mixing bowl.

8. Use a pastry cutter or your fingers to cut the cold, cubed butter into the flour mixture until it resembles coarse crumbs after adding it to the bowl.

9. The apples in the pie plate should be covered with the crumb topping.

10. Bake the apple pie for 45 to 50 minutes, or until the filling is bubbling and the crust is golden brown.

11. Before slicing and serving, allow the pie to cool for at least 30 minutes.

12. Sliced apples, sugar, cinnamon, nutmeg, salt, and flour for the filling should all be combined in a separate basin.

Peach Cobbler

Ingredients:

- 4 cups fresh or frozen sliced peaches
- 1/4 cup granulated sugar
- 1/4 cup brown sugar
- 1 tbsp cornstarch
- 1 tsp ground cinnamon
- 1/2 tsp ground nutmeg
- 1 tsp vanilla extract
- 1/4 cup unsalted butter, melted
- 1 cup all-purpose flour
- 1/4 cup granulated sugar
- 1/4 cup brown sugar
- 2 tsp baking powder

- 1/2 tsp salt

- 1 cup milk

Instructions:

1. A 9-inch square baking dish should be greased and the oven should be preheated to 375°F (190°C).

2. Toss the peaches in a large mixing dish with the sugars, cornstarch, cinnamon, nutmeg, vanilla essence, and melted butter. In the lined baking dish, distribute the peach mixture evenly.

3. For the cobbler batter, whisk together the flour, sugars, baking powder, and salt in a separate mixing basin.

4. Add the milk a little at a time while mixing the mixture to achieve smoothness.

5. The peaches in the baking dish should be covered with the cobbler batter.

6. For 45 to 50 minutes, or until the cobbler topping is golden brown and the peaches are bubbling, bake the peach cobbler.

7. At least 30 minutes should pass before serving the cobbler.

Carrot Cake with Cream Cheese Frosting

Ingredients:

(a.) For the cake:

- 2 cups all-purpose flour
- 2 tsp baking powder
- 1 tsp baking soda
- 1 tsp ground cinnamon
- 1/2 tsp ground ginger
- 1/4 tsp ground nutmeg
- 1/2 tsp salt
- 4 large eggs
- 1 1/2 cups granulated sugar

- 1 1/4 cups vegetable oil

- 1 tsp vanilla extract

- 3 cups grated carrots

- 1/2 cup chopped walnuts (optional)

(b.) For the cream cheese frosting:

- 8 oz cream cheese, softened

- 1/2 cup unsalted butter, softened

- 4 cups powdered sugar

- 1 tsp vanilla extract

Instructions:

1. Prepare two 9-inch cake pans with oil and preheat your oven to 350°F (175°C).

2. For the cake, combine the flour, baking powder, baking soda, cinnamon, ginger, nutmeg, and salt in a sizable mixing basin.

3. The eggs and sugar should be combined in a separate mixing dish and beaten until light and fluffy.

4. Whisking constantly, gradually incorporate the vegetable oil and vanilla essence into the egg mixture.

5. Just blend the dry components with the wet ones by folding them together.

6. Add the chopped walnuts and grated carrots (if using).

7. A toothpick inserted in the center of each cake should come out clean after baking for 30-35 minutes after evenly dividing the cake batter between the prepared cake pans.

8. The cakes should cool in the pans for ten minutes before being moved to a wire rack to finish cooling.

9. Cream the butter and cream cheese in a mixing bowl until smooth.

10. As you gradually mix in the powdered sugar, the frosting will become smooth and creamy.

11. Add the vanilla extract and stir.

12. Spread the cream cheese frosting over the top of one cake after it has completely cooled.

13. Spread extra frosting over the top of the cake before setting the second cake on top of it.

14. Optional: Add more chopped walnuts or shredded carrots to the cake's top for decoration.

15. Before serving, place the cake in the refrigerator to chill for at least 30 minutes.

Raspberry Cheesecake Bars

Ingredients:

(a.) For the crust:

- 1 1/2 cups graham cracker crumbs
- 1/4 cup granulated sugar
- 1/2 cup unsalted butter, melted

(b.) For the cheesecake filling:

- 16 oz cream cheese, softened
- 2/3 cup granulated sugar
- 2 large eggs
- 1 tsp vanilla extract
- 1/2 cup raspberry preserves
- Fresh raspberries, for topping

Instructions:

1. To begin, line an 8-inch square baking dish with parchment paper and preheat the oven to 350°F (175°C).

2. The graham cracker crumbs, sugar, and melted butter should all be thoroughly mixed together in a basin.

3. Using a glass with a flat bottom, press the crust mixture into the bottom of the baking dish as evenly as possible.

4. Cream cheese and sugar should be combined in a separate mixing dish and beaten until smooth and creamy.

5. Continue beating after adding the eggs and vanilla extract to get a smooth mixture.

6. Over the crust, pour the cheesecake mixture.

7. To achieve a marbled appearance, spoon the raspberry preserves over the cheesecake batter and gently swirl with a knife.

8. Bake the cheesecake for 35 to 40 minutes, or until it is firm.

9. Before putting the cheesecake in the refrigerator to chill for at least two hours, let it cool in the pan for 30 minutes.

10. The cheesecake should be refrigerated before being cut into bars and topped with a fresh raspberry before serving.

Chocolate Lava Cake

Ingredients:

- 4 oz unsalted butter

- 4 oz semi-sweet chocolate

- 1/2 cup granulated sugar

- 2 large eggs

- 2 large egg yolks

- 1/2 tsp vanilla extract

- 1/4 cup all-purpose flour

- Powdered sugar, for dusting

- Fresh berries, for serving (optional)

Instructions:

1. Grease four 6 ounce ramekins and preheat your oven to 425°F (218°C).

2. Melt the butter and chocolate together over low heat, stirring regularly, in a small saucepan.

3. Whisk the sugar, eggs, egg yolks, and vanilla extract until they are light and foamy in a mixing dish.

4. After adding the melted chocolate mixture, stir the egg mixture thoroughly.

5. The flour should be sifted on top of the chocolate mixture and whisked in briefly.

6. To evenly fill the ramekins, divide the batter.

7. The cakes should have the borders that are firm but the centers that are still a little jiggly after 12 to 14 minutes of baking when the ramekins are placed on a baking sheet.

8. The cakes should be taken out of the oven, cooled in the ramekins for five minutes, then placed on serving plates.

9. The cakes should be served with fresh berries, if preferred, and powdered sugar dusted on top.

Banana Bread with Walnuts

Ingredients:
- 2 cups all-purpose flour
- 1 tsp baking soda

- 1/2 tsp salt

- 1/2 cup unsalted butter, softened

- 1 cup granulated sugar

- 2 large eggs

- 1 tsp vanilla extract

- 3 ripe bananas, mashed

- 1/2 cup chopped walnuts

Instructions:

1. Grease a 9x5 inch loaf pan and preheat the oven to 350°F (175°C).

2. The flour, baking soda, and salt should all be thoroughly blended in a mixing dish.

3. Beat the butter and sugar together until they are light and fluffy in another mixing dish.

4. Once they are thoroughly mixed, add the eggs and vanilla extract.

5. Add the flour mixture gradually, stirring until barely blended.

6. Mash the bananas and add the walnuts, then stir in.

7. Fill the prepared loaf pan with the batter.

8. If you insert a toothpick into the center of the loaf, it should come out clean after 60 to 70 minutes of baking.

9. Prior to moving the banana bread to a wire rack to finish cooling, allow it to cool in the pan for 10 minutes.

10. Banana bread can be served warm or at room temperature. Slice and serve.

Tiramisu

Ingredients:

- 6 egg yolks

- 3/4 cup granulated sugar

- 2/3 cup whole milk
- 1 1/4 cups heavy cream
- 1/2 tsp vanilla extract
- 1/4 cup Marsala wine
- 8 oz mascarpone cheese
- 24 ladyfingers
- 1/2 cup strong coffee, cooled
- Cocoa powder, for dusting

Instructions:

1. The egg yolks and sugar should be combined in a mixing basin and whisked until light and foamy.

2. The milk should be heated in a small saucepan over medium heat until it just begins to simmer.

3. While continuously whisking, slowly incorporate the heated milk into the egg mixture.

4. When the mixture has thickened enough to coat the back of a spoon, pour it back into the saucepan and simmer it over low heat, stirring frequently.

5. Turn off the heat source and allow the custard to cool completely.

6. Beat the heavy cream, vanilla bean paste, and Marsala wine until stiff peaks form in a mixing basin.

7. Mascarpone cheese should be creamier and smoother after being beaten in another mixing dish.

8. Till the mascarpone cheese is thoroughly blended, gently fold the whipped cream into it.

9. Place the ladyfingers in a single layer in the bottom of a 9 x 13 inch baking dish after dipping them in the cooled coffee.

10. The ladyfingers should be covered with half of the mascarpone mixture.
11. Repeat the process with the remaining mascarpone mixture and a second layer of dipped ladyfingers.

12. Place the baking dish in the refrigerator for at least two hours or overnight. Cover with plastic wrap.

13. Before serving, sprinkle some cocoa powder on top of the tiramisu.

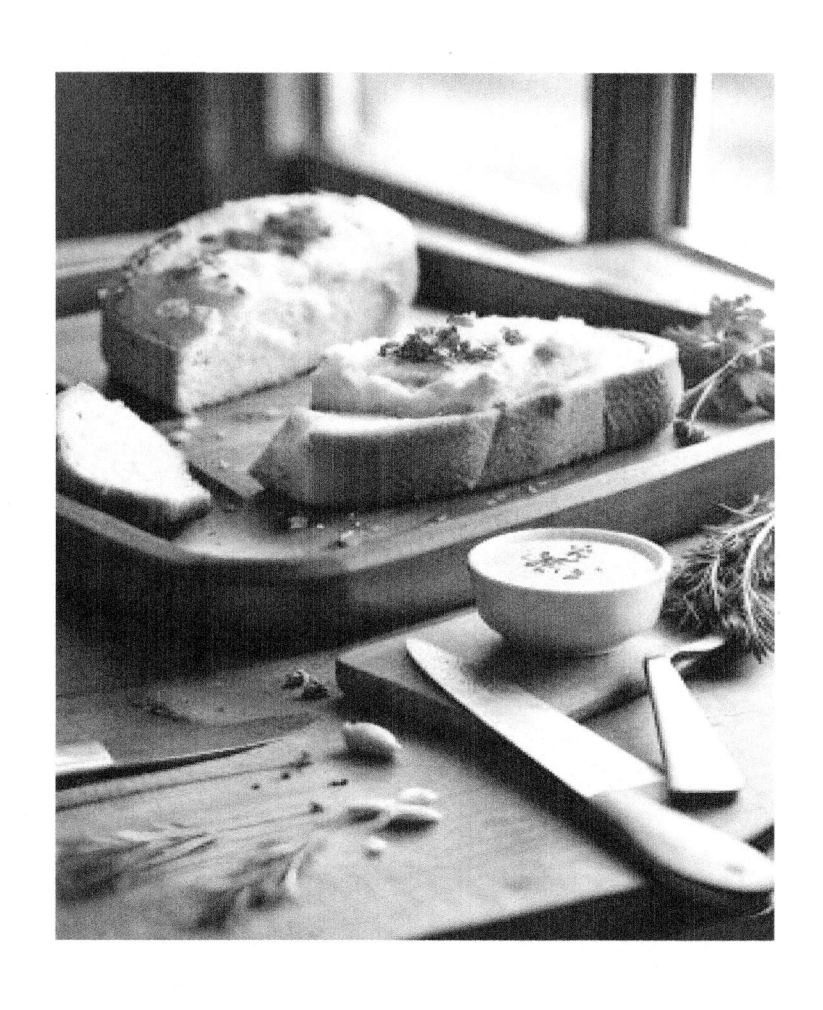

CONCLUSION

In conclusion, managing celiac illness can be difficult, particularly when it comes to preparing meals. However, a healthy lifestyle and scrumptious, nutrient-dense meals are achievable with the correct information and tools. With a variety of gluten-free recipes for breakfast, lunch, supper, snacks, and desserts, this cookbook for children with Celiac disease makes it simpler for parents and other caregivers to make sure their child is getting the nutrients they require without running the danger of ingesting gluten.

Parents can guarantee that their child is secure and healthy while still savoring a broad selection of delectable dishes by adhering to the guidelines for cooking and eating gluten-free. It's critical to keep in mind that having Celiac disease does not need giving up flavor or appreciation of food.

It's possible to construct a varied and fulfilling menu that meets the needs of people with Celiac disease because there are so many gluten-free products and recipe options available. Parents and other caregivers can feel assured that they can feed their children delicious, wholesome meals that are gluten-free with the help of this cookbook and other resources.

Continue your culinary explorations and test out some of the other gluten-free recipes on hand to make sure your youngster is receiving the finest nutrition while savoring a variety of delectable dishes. It is possible to live well with Celiac disease if you have the correct information, tools, and attitude.

Printed in Great Britain
by Amazon